WHITE GIRL IN YOGA PANTS

Stories of Yoga, Feminism, & Inner Strength

Melissa Scott

DEDICATION

For my babies--past, present, and future

AUTHOR'S NOTE

This book addresses topics that may be triggering to some readers. The author has placed warnings on chapters with potentially triggering material so that readers can make informed choices as they read.

TABLE OF CONTENTS

ABOUT THIS BOOK

This book is a love letter in three parts.

It is a love letter to the divine strength we all have inside of us. The unending, powerful, resilient strength that keeps us moving forward.

The first part is about how that strength shows up on the yoga mat. It includes stories about how I found my personal strength through yoga, how I came to teach and share those moments with my students and teacher trainees, and how the process of self-discovery continues to unfold for me.

The second part is about how strength shows up in society on a broader, more public scale. In these turbulent times fraught with divisive discourse, it's hard not to feel beaten down and discouraged. And so we must look for and celebrate the strength in our communities, in our convictions, and in each other.

The third part is about how strength shows up in life, in both the mundane and the extraordinary moments. It's about how we find our strength in the challenging times and celebrate it in the good times.

And so this is the journey. We start by looking at what's small and close to home, then widen our view, only to return back to the present and personal and apply the lessons we learned. From micro to macro and back again. Expand and contract. Ebb and flow.

Breathe in. Breathe out.

INTRODUCTION: YOU'RE STRONGER THAN YOU THINK YOU ARE

Shit happens.

Hard shit, good shit, depressing shit, funny shit, traumatic shit, inspiring shit, confusing shit. All kinds of shit.

Shit happens to us and around us every day. Some of it is our own doing; we make it happen. Some of it is totally outside of our control.

We all do our best to handle our shit. Sometimes we work ourselves to the bone to deal with it. Sometimes we crawl into bed and pull the covers over our head to avoid it. Sometimes we just put one foot in front of the other and try to do the next right thing.

Sometimes we take on other people's shit and try to manage it for them. (You should stop doing that, by the way.)

Sometimes we believe that we are defined by the shit that happens to us. Or that our shit makes us unlovable or not good enough. Or that we should be ashamed of it. We let those beliefs weaken and limit us. We feel depressed and anxious. We find unhealthy ways to deal with those feelings.

I know that because I've been there.

Like you, I've been through a lot of shit. I've had an eating disorder, been raped, been divorced, struggled with negative body image and crippling depression, found myself unexpectedly alone in my 30s and had to rebuild my life from scratch, dated unhealthy people and survived the subsequent break-ups, and managed health crises that threatened my livelihood and future.

In each of those situations, I could have chosen defeat.

And a lot of times I did. I gave into limiting beliefs about myself and what I deserved in life. I thought that I was no better than my shit.

But after a lot of therapy, a lot of yoga, a lot of stupid choices, a lot of self-help books, and a lot of conversations with some amazingly supportive friends, I learned something pretty radical about all the shit I've been through. One overarching truth about all of it.

I got through it.

Every time I thought I couldn't deal with this latest ordeal, I did. It might not have been pretty, but I managed and came out on the other side realizing that I'm so much stronger than I thought I was.

And you're stronger than you think you are, too.

You are not defined by your shit. You're bigger and stronger and better than it is. And, if you embrace the power you have inside you, you'll spend the rest of your life blowing your own mind at how strong and resilient and inspiring you are.

I see this on the yoga mat all the time. My students constantly do things they thought they'd never be able to. Headstands, arm balances, splits. For some people, just being able to touch their toes is a "wow" moment. I live for that, the look of euphoria and surprise on their faces when they spend a breath or two in a pose they thought was outside of their reach. Because I know that they're connecting with the power and potential they have inside them, and nothing feels better than that.

I know that feeling because that's what my practice has given me for almost 15 years. It's a constant reminder that I'm still moving, still capable, still growing. It's not always "wow" moments. Sometimes life is so overwhelming that just the act of showing up on my mat is worth celebrating. But that's the constant, reassuring whisper when I come to practice: "Hey, look, you're still here. You've still got this."

Believing in your own strength is addictive. It was for me. The more I did it, the more I wanted to. When I saw just how strong I can be, when I actually owned that belief, I started making really kick-ass decisions. I ate healthier and only exercised in ways that I loved, rather than punishing my body. I made better choices in relationships instead of settling for less than I deserved. I left a soul-crushing job in favor of dream-chasing self-employment that fulfills me like nothing else. And I dedicated myself to a life of travel and adventure that constantly pushes me outside of my comfort zone.

I want the same thing for you. I want you to get hooked on your own strength. I want you to be bold and take risks and trust yourself in everything you do.

I want you to see that you're better than your shit and the stories that came with it.

You're so much more than that.

And you're so much stronger than you think you are.

PART ONE:

Yoga

CHAPTER 1

HOW IT ALL STARTED

My earliest memories are defined by movement. Learning to do a cartwheel. Climbing the gigantic tree in my great-grandmother's backyard. Skipping across a rubber floor in pink shoes and tights. Chasing after fireflies in wet grass. Zipping down the highway on yet another family road trip. My earliest memories are in my body. Movement--both literal and metaphorical--is comfortable and natural to me. It's how I relate to the world.

During my childhood, my parents indulged almost any interest my brother and I had, so I dabbled in lots of things--gymnastics, art, piano. But dance my was my consistent love.

I started with pre-school jazz and tap classes, but fell head over heels in love with ballet. I loved the tutus, the buns, the shiny pink ribbons on pointe shoes. Mostly, I loved how moving gracefully felt like a superpower.

Ballet suited me more than other styles of dance, and even within my preferred discipline, I wasn't the most gifted. I struggled to jump and turn. I'm not a quick mover. But when the tempo slowed for an adagio sequence, I really shined. I appreciated the subtlety of quieter, more somber movement. Slow and graceful am I.

I was apprenticed to Montgomery Ballet in late elementary school. Apprenticeship is an old tradition in the dance world in which young dancers commit to training under experienced teachers. On a practical level, it means hours at the studio, back to back classes, and a whole lot of hair pins. My apprenticeship taught me the quiet beauty of dedication to practice.

In college, I was lucky enough to both attend a university with a thriving Dance program and nationally recognized professors, and to be on full academic scholarship, which allowed me to take electives and explore a variety of interests for free. I wasn't quite talented enough to major in dance, and I had other interests to pursue, but I enrolled in at least one dance class every semester to stay connected to my training. For the first time, I branched outside of ballet to explore jazz and modern dance. My body moved in new and exciting ways. It was a thrilling time to be in my skin.

Up to that point, I'd never given much thought to yoga. I was aware it existed, but I knew next to nothing about it.

I don't remember who first said to me, "You should try yoga." Most likely someone in my dorm who knew I danced and enjoyed moving. Growing up in the dance world gave me a certain fearlessness in my body, so I was willing to try almost any physical pursuit once.

There was only one yoga studio in Tuscaloosa, AL at the time. It was a tiny, one-room situation with office-style carpet and a pile of thin sticky mats. They offered student rates for only five dollars a class, which fit into my measly sophomore budget. The woman who ran it was a tiny, curly-haired Canadian who said the word "again" with a long "a" sound in the second syllable and played slow, ambient music as students arrived.

I was hooked the second I walked in the door.

It was so similar to my dance world, and yet so different. The same purposeful arrival, finding your space in the room, settling into physical practice. But it lacked the tension of dance class. There was no pressure to perform. I didn't have to get anything "right." No one ever told me to go back and do something again because I hadn't completed the correct form. I could check out and be guided in movements that suited my strengths, slow and graceful.

I probably would have kept doing yoga regardless, but the final moments of that first class solidified my lifelong commitment before I even stepped off my mat.

That first Savasana. The first time in my life I was allowed to rest, told to rest. No pressure to move or do or be anything in particular. Permission to be still for the first time.

The teacher laid an eye pillow on my face. The room settled into silence.

And I cried.

I can't even tell you now, all these years later, exactly what I cried about. Unnamed emotions welled up in my belly, distorting my face as I attempted to sob quietly. Wave after wave of emotion washed over me and spilled out through my eyes. Twenty years worth of something I couldn't identify came up, came out, and left.

In the midst of this intense release, part of my mind remained detached, observing. It was as though I was standing back and watching with objective curiosity, sort of a "Huh, isn't that interesting?" And in that detachment, I felt intense peace.

I have no idea what I cried about that day, other than a lifetime of hurts and sadness and the struggle of an eating disorder I wasn't ready to let go of yet. I knew that it felt good to release, and I knew I needed it. I soaked that eye pillow and felt no shame for it. I rolled up my mat and walked out into the sunshine feeling lighter than I ever had in my life.

I drove directly to TJ Maxx and bought a five dollar yoga mat. I walked next door to Barnes & Noble and bought a book of yoga poses. I don't remember consciously deciding to do these things, but rather was motivated by some other force, perhaps that objective observer inside me who entertained a deep curiosity about yoga. There was no question about buying these things and committing. This was a thing I needed to do.

As much as anyone can know at the age of 20, I knew I would do yoga for the rest of my life.

I spent that summer exploring the practice, both on my own and in class. At home, I rolled out my mat and opened my book and experimented with those pose and that pose, no real thought to sequencing, just a blissful play. In class, I was guided by teachers, told that everything that happened on my mat was okay, and encouraged to breathe.

It was a sweet and magical time in my life, those early months of yoga practice. I knew I was making a lifelong commitment to something, but I wasn't sure what that something was yet. I couldn't see yet the places yoga would take me, or the people it would connect me to. I couldn't guess that, a decade later, yoga would become my full-time job.

Those things weren't important for me to know yet. The practice gave me what I needed then, which was a safe space to release and explore. All I needed to know back then was just how good it felt to be still.

CHAPTER 2

WEIRDOS: THE ART OF LIVING YOUR YOGA

Admit it: Yoga made you weird.

Your friends comment on how different you are than you used to be. People laugh and roll their eyes when you talk. You've gotten used to getting strange looks and have accepted you probably will for the rest of your life.

Yeah, me too.

Practicing yoga changes you. First, your habits change. You start molding your schedule around your favorite classes and saying things like, "I can't stay out late. I have yoga in the morning."

Next, your relationship with your body changes. You start choosing foods that feel good to your body, which means you have to skip those late-night Taco Bell runs with friends. You may even cut out or cut down on socializing staples, like alcohol or caffeine, making you that water-drinking weirdo at the bar. And then, your relationships start to change. As you honor yourself more, you start setting boundaries where you haven't before. You approach a previously volatile relationship with more compassion. And you even start to apply that whole "We are all one" thing people always talk about.

Living your yoga takes some courage. You either know going in or figure out very quickly that it's going to rock some boats. People feel comfortable with the status quo, and when you start changing things in your own life, it will affect theirs, too. They may react from a place of fear, which can come across as judgment, anger, mocking, or withdrawal. To stay strong and compassionate, and to continue to live your yoga in the face of those responses is a major act of bravery.

I've heard some amazing weirdo stories from yogi friends who fearlessly live their practice and aren't afraid to show it. One student had an outdoor wedding in the summer. She didn't want to get overheated in her wedding dress, so when she got warm, she did a cooling shitali breath right there at her wedding reception. If you want to stand out as a breath-loving yogi, shitali--with its rolled-tongue inhales--is definitely the way to go.

Another friend and fellow teacher feels passionate about compost, so she took her compost worms to her son's elementary classroom to teach them about the benefits of composting. While other parents might think she's a little strange, the kids loved it. She joyfully embraces the nickname "Worm Mom."

I remember marking myself as a total weirdo when I briefly lived in Chicago after college. I took public transit on a daily basis, and at the time I was really getting into the idea of all people as a manifestation of God's love. One of my daily practices was to thank my bus driver any time I got off at my stop. One day, I remember hearing some girls laughing behind me, saying, "Who thanks the bus driver?! It's not like they did anything for you!" But to my yoga brain, they did. And more importantly, they were a human, just like me, worthy of acknowledgement and respect, even on the cold streets of Chicago.

I've heard yogis talk about how difficult it was to become the only non-drinking member in their party-loving group of friends, or how other parents judged their yoga-based child-rearing practices. Cookouts are constant challenges as family and friends struggle to understand and accommodate our different diets. It would be easy to hide our yoga-based practices. Easy, but not authentic. And one of yoga's great lessons is how to truly be yourself. Your freaky, weird, worm-loving, human-acknowledging, public-shitali-breathing self.

CHAPTER 3

YOGA LOVE

It was love at first meeting. That kind of sudden, deep, knock-your-socks off love that changes everything. I was twenty years old and walked away from that first encounter knowing this would be a lifelong thing. This would be the kind of relationship I'd write a book about years later. I had found The One.

I'm talking, of course, about yoga. The great love of my life.

Yoga and I fell passionately in love from the first moment we met. Our first encounter was at a tiny, one-room studio in a strip mall in the college town where I went to school. The room was smoky from incense, and the handful of regulars comfortably chatted and joked. It was the yoga equivalent of meeting in a dive bar. After that day, I changed everything to spend more time with my new love. I changed my schedule, my wardrobe, even my friends to make room for this exciting new relationship.

Like all relationships, the honeymoon phase didn't last forever. (Don't let the Twilight movies fool you; it never does.) Soon yoga and I settled into a comfortable routine. The butterflies faded, but the relationship was still happy, sweet, and fulfilling. Yoga was there for me when I went to bed at night, giving me soothing restorative poses and peaceful savasana to relax me to sleep. It was there for me in the morning, giving me invigorating Sun Salutations to energize and strengthen me for the day. It was there for me during stressful times, during happy times, and during those just-getting-through-the-day times. For years, we carried on in committed bliss.

Like any relationship we eventually hit some bumps in the road. The love was still there, but the passion was gone. The poses became routine, the practice monotonous. I came to my mat more out of obligation than desire. And one day, after a particularly dull practice, when I was struggling to get through even the most basic poses, it hit me.

Yoga and I needed a break.

I was ashamed to admit it, but there it was. The Truth. I needed space from yoga, and if my practice could have talked, it probably would have admitted it needed space from me, too.

So in a bittersweet moment, I rolled up my mat and tucked it into a corner, where I knew it might stay a while. In my memory, I actually shed a tear or two, knowing that it would probably be awhile before we saw each other again. But with resolve, I walked away, sure that I would come back, but unsure of when.

For the next six months, I did the mind-body equivalent of dating around. I took pilates classes. I lifted weights. I spent hours on cardio machines at the gym. I took a stab (and failed miserably) at running. I meditated more. I read about Taoism and Tantra. A little of this, a little of that. I flirted and explored. Until finally I found myself, on a gloriously sunny Sunday afternoon, mat in hand, back in the vinyasa class that had long been a favorite before yoga and I hit our rough patch.

I chose my space. I set down my water bottle. I unrolled my mat, taking a moment to tenderly smooth down its curled up edges. "I missed you, baby," I said. "Will you please take me back?"

That class was one of the stretchiest, breathiest, most joyous practices I'd ever had. It felt like slipping back into the arms of a long-lost lover. Familiar, loving, safe. I wondered why I had been away so long, but knew I could never have had that feeling if yoga and I hadn't taken a break from each other.

Not long after that day, I enrolled in a teacher training, which for me felt like the equivalent of asking yoga to marry me. On the day of my teacher training graduation, I felt like I was saying "I do" to my practice. And we've been happily committed ever since.

That's not to say we don't have hard times. Some days I still look at my mat and say, "Seriously? You again? I'm so not in the mood for what you have to offer." But we always make up. My practice always forgives my bad attitude and less-than-open heart, and always welcomes me back, the same generous, nurturing, invigorating love it's always been.

A few years ago, yoga and I had a renaissance of sorts. My body got stronger and my spirit a little more adventurous, which opened up a whole new world of arm balances and inversions. My practice and I felt like the old married couple who had fallen back in love with each other and started taking wildly daring vacations, recapturing the spirit of their youthful, honeymoon days.

Now is a beautiful time in our relationship. But I know this phase won't last. I know there will be hard times, and there may even come a time when we need space from each other again. But I always try to apply the lessons of my practice and just stay in the moment, enjoying where we are. Right here, right now. Together.

CHAPTER 4

THE JOURNEY TO TEACHING

Trigger Warning: Eating Disorders

I'm a pathological leader.

I can't get involved with something without eventually taking on a leadership role. I'm never content to sit and participate. I simply have to get involved and put my stamp on something somehow. I'll offer to organize events or oversee the money or--more often than not--be president of the whole damn organization in which I take on too much responsibility and end up burning myself out.

After I started doing yoga, it was only a matter of time before I started teaching it.

There was so little information about yoga in Alabama when I first started practicing in 2003. There was only one tiny studio in Tuscaloosa, and only one or two in Birmingham, the "big city" (population: under 1 million at that time) just an hour up the road. The internet was not yet the information overload it is now, Facebook had just been invented and was populated exclusively by college students, and social media as we know it today didn't exist. Yoga classes were huge in places like California and New York, where Power Flow was having its heyday, but in Alabama, we were excited about getting six or eight people together for a few poses.

Being the 20-year little old go-getter I was, I'm sure I asked one of my yoga teachers how a motivated yogi goes about becoming a yoga teacher. At the time, I assumed you had to practice for many years before pursuing a teacher training program. And back then, that was certainly more the norm than it is now. I knew I was interested in pursuing my 200-hour teacher training at some point, but I put those ambitions on the back burner while I focused on school, graduate school ambitions, and enjoying my practice as a support to my dance training.

In the Spring of 2005, my life hit two major turning points. First, I was accepted to a highly competitive Ph.D. program at the University of Illinois-Chicago. Second, I sustained a major injury in a dance class that left me in a boot cast for a while and ended my ballet career. (If you've never heard your own ankle make a sound like a gunshot, have you ever really lived?) In one second, dance was out of my life, leaving a void for movement and self-expression.

In the August of 2005, only 22 and still rehabbing from my injury, I moved to Chicago to begin graduate school. I found a cute studio apartment in Wrigleyville, familiarized myself with the public transportation system, and bought all my books for the semester. I then proceeded to spiral into the darkest period of my life.

Chicago was too much. It was too big and crowded, and too different from home. I knew no one in the city except classmates I had just met. And so, when I started to have mysterious health and neurological issues that had me in and out of various emergency rooms, I had no one to lean on. I missed class often, which my gracious professors excused with offers to work with me. I became massively depressed, spending all of my free time alone in my tiny studio apartment listening to NPR podcasts on repeat. And, most devastating of all, I gave in completely to the eating disorder I had been fighting off an on for most of the last decade.

My weight loss was rapid. Classmates and professors commented on it. I excused it by saying it was related to my other health problems, which they knew I was having. My clothes hung off of me, and I was freezing all the time. As Fall became Winter, my exposed bones ached with cold. I felt empty and light, like I could evaporate at any time.

One day, some time between Halloween and Thanksgiving, I glanced into a store window as I walked down the street. For a split second, I thought someone had neglected to take down a spooky skeleton decoration.

But then I realized, Oh my God, that's my reflection.

Not everyone who struggles with an eating disorder has this kind of "aha" moment, and I'm not sure why the Universe chose to give me one then and there on the streets of Chicago. But I know for certain that seeing my reflection that day and the abject terror it inspired saved my life.

When I went home for Thanksgiving a couple of weeks later, I tearfully broke down on my Dad's couch. I told him I couldn't do it, that I was sick and scared and needed to come home. I didn't say that I was afraid I might die, but that was the undercurrent of my words. He agreed to come rescue me.

Prideful, I insisted on finishing out the semester. Even though I wasn't going to finish my program, I needed to show myself that I could accomplish something in the face of all that turmoil. Miraculously, and perhaps due to the pity and compassion of my professors, I finished the semester with all A's.

The day after my I submitted my final paper, my Dad arrived at O'Hare Airport. By the next day, we had everything I owned packed in a UHaul. We pulled away just as the snow began to fall.

My father and I have had our ups and downs in our relationship, but I know for certain that he loves me. And I know that because that night, he drove for hours through a blizzard in a Uhaul with his sick and broken daughter, knowing that he was saving her life. As we drove south on I-65, the snowfall got heavier, and at times we couldn't see much past the nose of the truck. I asked him several times if he wanted to stop, but he said no, we'll stop once we get out of this bad weather. And so on we crept, in a slow motion emergency evacuation toward home.

By the time we got to a cheap motel outside of Louisville around 1am, I knew we were going to be okay. And more importantly, I knew I was going to live.

I landed back in Birmingham shortly before Christmas, unemployed, living with my mother, and physically weakened by illness and eating disorder. The next few months were about rehabbing and reclaiming my life. I landed a full-time job at a mental health facility. I took a play therapy class for fun at the local university that led me to enroll in the Master's in Counseling program. I met and started dating the man who would become my husband a few years later. I ate and gained a little weight and saw a therapist and got stronger. And I went to as many yoga classes as I could while maintaining a consistent home practice.

By the Fall of 2007, I was strong, healthy, and happy. I had a solid year of eating disorder recovery behind me was thriving in my graduate program. The deeper I dove into the theory and practice of Counseling, the more room I saw for applying yoga to therapeutic practices. I began talking to my professors and classmates about my ideas for using yoga with clients.

I don't remember consciously deciding I was ready to do yoga teacher training. All I remember is coming to in front of my computer at work deep in a Google search for yoga teacher trainings in the Southeast. There were no programs in Alabama at that time, so I searched for programs in cities I could drive to easily: Nashville, Atlanta, Charlotte.

Chattanooga.

There she was, on the website of a studio I'd never heard of. Petite with bangs, sparkly blue eyes, and the brightest, most disarming smile I'd ever seen. Dolly Stavros, from Charlotte, NC, leading a yoga teacher training in Chattanooga.

Oh, good! I thought. Here's my teacher training.

I'm not one to make rash decision, but occasionally I encounter a situation and know exactly what I need to do, and I jump. And in this case, I was ready to jump.

I emailed Dolly and asked if we could talk on the phone before I registered for training. She called me the next day, and we talked for about 15 minutes. As soon as we got off the phone, I wrote her a check out of my student loan money for the full tuition amount, booked an apartment to stay in for the first module, and started telling people about my exciting new plans. I was ready to breeze my way into this exciting new chapter.

I had no idea teacher training would make me deal with literally all of my shit.

Here's the thing about yoga teacher training: It's raw. It's vulnerable. You're locked in a room for 200 hours with a bunch of strangers, doing and talking about this life-changing practice that you're still trying to get your head around, and then standing up in front of those people to use your own voice to tell them how to use their bodies and how to breathe and how to connect spiritually, and hold on a second while I do some breathing exercises into this paper bag, y'all just hang out in Child's Pose.

I don't know anyone who hasn't confronted their "stuff" in the face of all that vulnerability. Teacher trainings are notorious cry-fests. There's a morbid joke in some circles that every teacher training program in the country is responsible for at least one divorce a year. The truth is that yoga is transformational, and going deeper with it leads to deeper transformation. And to transform deeply, we have to look deeply at the things that hold us back.

At the time I started teacher training, my single greatest struggle in life was perfectionism. A high-achieving nature combined with nearly two decades of classical dance training left me with little room for error. I put extraordinary pressure on myself to do, say, and be all the right things. I heavily edited my interactions with people and would cry for days if I thought I'd said or done the wrong thing. That toxic pressure on myself had led to my eating disorder; I believed if I could just look perfect enough, I would be free from criticism and wholly lovable.

All this perfectionism made me really good at faking it. I'd been the president of every club I joined in college and had developed a faux confidence that masked my deep insecurities. I would smile and charm and impress people with my intelligence, and then disappear into my own head and castigate myself for not being good enough, vowing to do even better and be even more perfect next time.. I showed up to the first day of training prepared to wow everyone with how "good" I was at standing up and speaking in front of people. I was prepared to be the star of the the training and do everything just right.

Little did I know, Dolly had a gift for peeling back people's defenses and exposing the rawness inside. On the very first day of training, with no warning and no preparation, Dolly made us lead the entire group through three Sun Salutations, knowing how terrible and awkward we would be at them. We did exercises that involved staring into a peer's eyes for five minutes without speaking. We had group conversations about vulnerability and being authentic as an inherent part of teaching yoga.

It's hard to imagine anything that could have challenged me more at that point in my life. I had to come to terms with the fact that I had lived a long time as a performative shell of a person. I had very little real sense of self, and I recognized in teacher training an opportunity to build an authentic "me," free of the pressure to do and say everything just right.

As my perfectionistic walls crumbled, my teacher training experience unfolded before me with grace, healing, and openness. I let myself cry as I shared my writing assignments. I was silly and laughed at my mistakes. Not usually one for affection, I let myself be touched and hugged, and on the last day of training, crawled into a giant cuddle puddle with my fellow trainees, recognizing that I had allowed them deep into my heart and never wanted to let them go. I was finally open to being my real self, and I finally had an idea of who that self would be.

A few days after graduating my teacher training program, I went to my favorite studio to take my favorite Sunday afternoon class, still uncertain how or when teaching would unfold for me. There was a sign on the door that said "Class cancelled. Apologies for any inconvenience." Along with that sign, the keys to the studio hung in the door lock, as though someone had locked the door, then absentmindedly walked away.

I pulled out my cell phone and called the studio owner. I left him a message to let him know I had his keys and would keep them safe until I could get them back to him.

He called me back a few hours later, grateful for rescuing his keys and apologetic that the class was cancelled.

"I wish I'd known," I said. "I just got back from teacher training. I would have prepared something."

"Do you want that class?" he asked. "That teacher quit today, and I don't have anyone to take it. It's yours if you want it."

I looked down at the studio key in my hand. The key that was in the door. I heard the Universe laugh gently at me, as it often does when it nudges me in the direction of the next great thing. Of course I was nervous about the idea of teaching actual people in an actual studio. But I had two choices: I could let my perfectionism, which I had spent so much time in the last year fighting, drag me down once again. Or I could say yes and open up to the journey yoga teaching could take me on.

"I'd love to!" I said brightly, internally acknowledging and externally masking the intense terror I felt, recognizing that this was my next great test in being vulnerable and open, and commending myself for the courage to say yes to this next big adventure.

"I'll be there next week!"

CHAPTER 5

LETTER TO MY STUDENTS

Dear Yogi,

We've known each other for a while now. Or maybe we just met this week. You've been coming to my class regularly for months. Or maybe you drop in from time to time when you can. Or maybe today was our first time to practice together. Whatever the circumstances, I get the pleasure of sharing yoga with you. But we don't always have a lot of time to talk. You're rushing in from your busy life, and I'm rushing out to mine, or there might be a class before or after that we have to clear out for. We don't always get to connect in person. But there are some things I want you to know.

I think about you a lot. Whenever I discover a nugget of wisdom or have an idea for a new sequence, I wonder if you'll like it. When I try a new pose in my own practice, I think about how I might break it down to teach it to you. I look up quotes on the internet hoping they will inspire you during those hard, sweaty moments. I wonder if you'll come to class today, and if I haven't seen you in a while, I wonder how you're doing. You're always in the back of my mind, and I'm always excited to see you again.

You inspire me. The fact that you show up to yoga, that you're so courageous in the work that you do, rocks my world. When you tell me about books you're reading, meditations you're practicing, or retreats you're going on, it inspires me to be a better, more devoted yogi, too. The quotes you share with me, the way you laugh at yourself when you fall out of a pose, the way you overcome your fear to try that freaky new arm balance—none of that goes unnoticed. I take your courage and excitement home with me, and it energizes me, too.

I believe in you. Those arm balances and inversions I talk you into? The ones where you look at me like I'm crazy for even suggesting it? I believe you can do them. I wouldn't suggest them if I didn't. In fact, I believe you're so much stronger than you think you are. (Maybe you've heard me say that before?) You're a lot braver, too. You're capable of so much, and it's exciting to share those moments with you when you realize it, too.

It's an honor to be a part of your life. The little conversations we have before and after class—the ones where you tell me about your break-up, your new job, how the tomatoes in your garden are growing—are an incredible honor. You let me into parts of your life and let me share your joy and pain. I'm humbled that you want to share those things with me.

I'm only human. I get nervous before class sometimes, wondering if you'll like the sequence I have planned today. I stumble over my words and forget what we did from the right leg to the left. I've kicked over water bottles, walked into space heaters, and forgotten the names of the most common poses. Sometimes teaching is an exercise in being okay with looking like a fool. I hope you forgive me, and I hope my humanness helps give you permission to be human, too.

I'm thankful for you. Without you, I couldn't do the thing I love to do most. Without you, there would be no class to teach. Without you, I wouldn't be able to spend time every week in beautiful community with other yogis. I'm always so glad to see you walk in the door before class, and I'm so glad to get to share this yoga practice with you.

I pray for you. At the end of every class, while you're resting in Savasana, I say a prayer for you. I pray that you will be peaceful and at ease, that your life will be full of joy and purpose, and that you will always feel full of gratitude. I don't know for sure if it makes a difference in your life, but it seems like the least I can do, after all you've done for me.

When I became a yoga teacher, I had no idea how much it would fill my life up with amazing people. The yoga is life-changing, of course. But the people—the community that's created around the yoga—for me, is the best part of all.

Thanks for coming.

Namaste,
Melissa

CHAPTER 6

MAKING TEACHER TRAINING

"I'll love you forever. I'll like you for always. As long as
I'm living, my baby you'll be."

- I'll Love You Forever, Robert Knapp

I really, really did not want to create a yoga teacher training. I fought it for a year. A year in which I sat around lamenting that no one in Birmingham was leading a teacher training like the one I went through, one that focused on self, personal growth, and living into the role of Teacher. I sat around lamenting it long enough, in fact, that it finally occurred to me: Oh, shit, it's gotta be me.

Like I said, I'm a pathological leader. If I see a thing needs to be done, I will do that thing. But the thought of leading a teacher training was uniquely intimidating. Only one other training existed in Birmingham, led by a charismatic teacher who had been teaching in town for as long as any local yogi could remember. Ashtanga was king in our yoga scene at that time, with most folks seeming to believe that everyone needed to be trained in the Primary Series

23

in order to teach. With my Core Strength Vinyasa training and wave-like motions on the mat, I was an outlier and an oddball in my home community. It felt borderline sacrilegious to offer another training, and I worried about stepping on well-respected toes. But I couldn't get the idea out of my head. Something was missing in the yoga landscape of my hometown, and I felt called to be the one to fill that gap.

In reality, it was a terrible time for me to take on such a huge project. I was smack in the middle of a divorce and processing the fear of being completely on my own for the first time in my life. I had a secure but soul-sucking job as a therapist at an eating disorder treatment clinic and was happily teaching yoga on the side. I had a steady following that certainly wasn't large enough to justify leading an entire 200-hour training. And yet, the thought persisted.

In another sense, it was a perfect time for me to take on a life-changing new project. In my fear and grief over the end of my marriage, I needed a new goal to fixate on. Teacher training was a handhold just barely within my reach that I could use to pull myself into a new chapter of life. This is my pattern: I always direct the energy of heartbreak into passion projects. I don't know if it's sublimation, healthy coping, or a little of both, but my proudest creations have been birthed out of my deepest sadnesses. And this was certainly a time of deep sadness.

I kicked the idea around for a few weeks while my ex-husband packed his things and my house gradually emptied out. I kept the idea to myself as it clanged around in my head, ever-present, like an eager child asking to be born. I finally let the idea spill to my friend Carla Jean on a girls' road trip yoga weekend as we sat in a Whole Foods in Chattanooga, coincidentally--or perhaps poetically--just blocks from where I'd completed my own 200-hour training.

"I'm thinking about leading a teacher training," I said, sheepishly.

"I'd sign up," she said, without missing a beat or looking up from her salad.

Well, I'd at least have one person, I thought.

And just like that, I became a teacher trainer.

Developing a 200-hour teacher training is no small task, and Yoga Alliance--the governing body for yoga teaching certifications--is notoriously picky about approving new programs. For weeks, I poured myself into curriculum development and planning. Spreadsheets took over my life. I spent hours on the couch honing each section, planning the schedule, and creating marketing materials. I poured my heart and soul into it, crafting the training I wanted to see in the world, one that combined everything I loved about yoga, teaching, psychology, and the personal journey within. When the time finally came to announce the training on social media in August of 2013, I felt like I was launching a rocket. I hovered my cursor over the "post" button and thought, 3… 2… 1… blast off.

Applications began to trickle in. (True to form, Carla Jean got hers to me by the end of business on the day I announced.) By Christmas, I had enough people signed up to know I'd be able to pay my bills for a year, allowing me to walk away from my soul-sucking therapist job and devote myself to teaching yoga full-time. Years of contemplation and months of work added up to an experience that changed my life completely. By the time I gathered with my 21 trainees for the first time in March of 2014, I was ready and open to this new chapter.

And so we dove in, beginning with the history of yoga and moving onward from there. We explored philosophy and chakras, anatomy and poses, and the complex realities of standing in front of people to share this thing you love so much. Every day of training was a lifetime unto itself. We set intentions, we meditated, we did asana practice. We discussed things in small groups and as a larger whole. Inside jokes popped up and flourished, until by the end of training, we were practically speaking our own language. Along the way, through some mysterious alchemic formula I haven't quite parsed out yet, they learned how teach the practice of yoga.

I knew leading people through the process of becoming a yoga teacher would be incredible and satisfying, but I was totally unprepared for how much I would fall in love with them. I had no idea how much joy it would bring me to see them come together as a group, to love one another so much that they lay with heads in each other's laps to listen to lectures, to carry their friendships out into the world, beyond the walls of teacher training. I had no idea how full my heart would feel at the end of each weekend, seeing them make tangible progress forward toward their goals. I had no idea how deep into my heart their sweet spirits would burrow, taking up permanent residence in the vast spectrum of People I Will Love Forever.

A lot of life unfolds in that room over the course of nine months. We laugh a lot. We talk about yoga. We cry. Every year, somebody gets divorced; somebody gets pregnant; somebody gets a new job; somebody gets married; somebody tells a story about their life they've never shared before. It's an honor to walk through that much life with people, to a degree I struggle to put into words. Over time, their stories fall away, and I see only the pure Goodness within them. As people experience anxiety and joy and fear and sadness and gratitude and all the other emotions one may feel during a life-changing process, I get to witness the very essence of Namaste: The divine light in me honors the divine light in you. They are all Divine Lights to me.

I joke with my trainees that one of the benefits of teacher training is that graduates get me for life, and this is more true than they know. After they bestow upon me the great honor of getting to lead them for nine months, I am devoted to them forever. I will always make time to talk with them, text with them, meet them for coffee, whatever they need of me. They don't realize how much they add to my life. There are tough days when the only thing that keeps me moving is knowing I'll be with them again soon, laughing and moving and diving deep into the mysteries of Self and Practice. Nothing in the world cracks my heart as wide open as being with my trainees. I hope my legacy is how much I love them.

Last year, I got the devastating news that it's very unlikely I'll ever be able to have children of my own. I mourned and grieved and tried to process it the best I could. I was never completely sold on the idea of having children, but I also never expected to have that decision forcibly taken from me, either. Just weeks after receiving that news, I was back in the training room. As my trainees laid down for their first Savasana of the weekend, my heart sprung a leak, and great, big tears flowed down my cheeks. Their peacefulness was almost more than I could bear; I felt like a mother watching her child sleep. Except I had 20 of them, and they chose me.

I don't always buy into the "Everything happens for a reason" school of thought, but in that moment, it seemed to me that perhaps the reason I wasn't meant to have children is because I get to have them. I get to have those moments of witnessing their development and holding their hands for a while, encouraging them to grow and discover more of the world. If that's how I'm meant to nurture people in this lifetime, it's far more than I deserve.

This thing I created is bigger than me. What started as a compulsory message from the Universe and a distraction from grief has grown into the defining experience of my life. I am a better person for having said yes to the grand adventure of leading people through teacher training and opening my heart to loving them fully. When the first weekend in March rolls around every year, all I can do is step into the room and allow myself to get swept up in the process. I don't claim to be an expert in anything other than loving the people put in front of me in that room every year, but that is something I plan to do for the rest of my life.

I'll love them forever. I'll like them for always. As long as I'm living, my babies they'll be.

CHAPTER 7

BODY COMMENTS IN YOGA

Trigger Warning: Eating Disorders, Body Image, Body Comments

"Oh, and I have a six-pack now. I need to show you what poses I've been doing. You could get one, too!"

I almost choke on my pad woon sen.

Wait... what?, I think.

Let me back up...

I'm having dinner with a fellow yoga teacher at my favorite Thai place. We've spent the last 45 minutes talking about meditation, breath, the transformative power of yoga, and where we are in our respective yoga journeys. It's been an inspiring and energizing conversation. Then suddenly, without my consent and between bites of spicy noodles, we've taken the hard left turn into BodyTalksville.

Unfortunately, this is not the story of a single conversation with a single yogi. This has happened dozens of times in my yoga career, with dozens of people. The abrupt shift from the spiritual to the physical. From the internal to the external. That sudden, jarring, unfortunate reiteration that, according to Western society, women are expected to focus obsessively on perfecting their external appearance, to the exclusion of other pursuits.

Every time this happens, I feel a little betrayed. I came to yoga almost 15 years ago, deeply engrossed in an eating disorder. My behaviors spanned the gamut from restricting to compulsive over-exercising to drunken binge-eating. My relationship with food was chaotic, and my relationship with my body was abysmal after decades of dance training and a cacophony of "not good enough" messages about my physical appearance. I was 20 years old and totally unaware of how desperate I was for something different. I went to a yoga class at the suggestion of a dorm mate. During the final relaxation, I cried tears that seemed to come from deep inside my belly. I walked out of the class feeling lighter and more hopeful than I had been in my entire life. Though I continued to struggle with food and body image for several years, that day was the beginning of the end of the power my eating disorder had over me.

Because yoga has always been my safe haven from body judgments, I take it personally whenever a fellow yogi injects a body comment into the conversation. Dude, this is my safe space. Take your implied judgment and adherence to social norms elsewhere, please. Nama-freakin'-ste. What's so upsetting about these comments is that they're often veiled in pseudo-empowering language or spiritual overtones. My friend with the six-pack talks about how "strong" it feels despite being visibly underweight. Another friend talks about needing to work on the block in her second chakra so she can flatten her stomach. Others conveniently go on "cleanses" or "detox diets" just before swimsuit season. It's as if draping self-improvement language over these behaviors makes it any different than the crash-dieting and body-bashing I did in my teens and early twenties. It's hard for me not to hear this talk as anything other than dressed up body hate.

I came to yoga to find freedom from body hate. Not to flatten my stomach, but to radically, fully accept it in all it's Buddha-ness. It's taken me ten years, but I finally almost-kinda love the way the area below my belly button sticks out like a pouty lower lip. It's magazine-perfect, but it's mine, dammit. And I've fought long and hard for this much peace with it. To say glibly that a few extra poses on my mat would rid me of my God-given pooch is to dismiss all that hard internal work, to say that the tears in my therapist's office and the choked-down, just-gotta-get-through-it meals were meaningless. Because the whole time I could have done a few extra crunches or Boat poses and not had to bother with all that silly self-acceptance. I could be someone else's definition of perfect rather than my own definition of good enough. Understandably, this is a yucky prospect.

But at some point, I have to return to my yogi mindfulness and compassion. I recognize that not everyone came to yoga for the reasons I did. Yes, it does feel great to witness your body transform, and some people do yoga for that reason. Is their reason any less valid than mine? Of course not. Selfishly, I can hope that those people will shift their focus to the profound self-acceptance that I sought and found through yoga. But it's not my place to want that for them, nor is it my place to project my path onto theirs.

Everyone who practices yoga will experience a transformation of some kind. Part of my work has been to accept myself exactly as I am. The other part has been to accept others exactly as they are, wherever they may be in their process. Thanks to yoga, when I hear a friend exclaim over their new-found six-pack, I'm able to place a loving hand on my own belly, smile, and--genuinely--say, "I'm so happy for you."

CHAPTER 8

ALIGNMENT AS A BODY IMAGE ISSUE

Trigger Warning: Body Image

I'll never forget the day in teacher training Carol realized that her toes don't point the same direction as her knees.

It happened during our anatomy weekend, and we were exploring the variety of ways skeletons can differ from each other.

Carol felt liberated. "Everyone tells you to point your toes forward in Crescent Lunge, but when I do that, my knee falls in. So teachers try to correct that, but then my toes turn out. I thought I was just doing it all wrong!"

I thought I was just doing it wrong.

I hear this from students over and over again. Their bodies can't conform to alignment cues they've heard from teachers hundreds of times, so they assume there's something wrong with them. They fight with their bodies to create the shape they think they're supposed to be in. It doesn't work, so they get frustrated and feel bad. In some cases, they might limit their practice or stop practicing altogether, assuming they're just not "good" at yoga.

Alignment conversations are tricky. So much of what we know--or think we know--about proper asana alignment was handed down from venerable teachers of the previous century. Some yogis have an almost fanatical adherence to what their gurus taught.

31

Therein lies the problem: Those yoga teachers were wise and inspiring, but they weren't anatomists. In fact, they learned to teach in a time when we knew a fraction of what we know about the body today.

Old ideas about anatomy and physiology persist in yoga teachers' cues. For example, on the very barest of surfaces, "locking the knee" would seem to straighten and stabilize the standing leg in any balancing pose, so it's understandable that this cue found its way into some teachers' dialogue. More recent research tells us, however, that locking the knee might stabilize the leg in the moment, but it cuts off blood flow, causing potential tissue damage, and sets the knee up for injury long-term. A more effective and anatomy-conscious cue would be to gently lift the muscles around the knee to stabilize the joint. The difference is subtle, and many yoga teachers lack the anatomical confidence to make that distinction, so they fall back on easier shorthand cues like "lock the knee."

There are countless other examples of lazy or ineffective cues. One that irks me is to turn the back foot 45 degrees in Warriors 1 and 2. The angle of that foot rotation starts at the hip, and hip socket configuration varies widely from person to person. Some yogis ideal rotation might be 45 degrees, but others' might be anywhere from 60 to 30 degrees, with outliers even beyond that range. So why do yoga teachers insist that 45 degrees is the correct rotation? And for the student for whom 60 degrees is a more comfortable, less injurious angle, do we give them permission to be true to their unique body? Or do we enforce an arbitrary standard because our teachers told us to?

One of the most insidious examples of ineffective cuing--especially in the Ashtanga and Vinyasa traditions--is to "square the hips forward" in Warrior 1. Because the back heel is rotated in toward the midline, the pelvis is anchored in place in an externally rotated position. It's impossible for most people (again, with a few outlier exceptions) to square the hips forward without putting downward, shirring pressure on the knee joint--which is physically uncomfortable at best and injurious at worst--and even then, the hip points can never actually be "square." I've heard countless students claim they "hate" Warrior 1 because "I can't square my hips." Of course they can't; it's an anatomical impossibility. So why, then, do teachers insist on repeating these tired, injurious cues in class after class.

When I question teachers about their cuing, they most often get a wide-eyed look and say, "Well, that's what my teacher taught me, so..." Less often, they become defensive and give answers that suggest it's borderline sacrilege to question these established teachings. Let me be clear and say I don't wish to take anything away from our teachers of the last century. They gave us the practice. In many ways, their teachings are as important and relevant today as they were 50 to 100 years ago. But times and bodies have changed, and today's teachers are clinging to a severely outdated understanding of alignment.

When this particular understand of alignment was developed, asana was primarily taught to boys and young men in a time when life was generally more active. People walked more to get around, and food required more effort and energy to obtain than it generally does today. The bodies receiving this asana instruction were very different than the current typical yoga practitioner in the West, who is more likely to be female, have a sedentary or semi-sedentary job, and drives or rides public transportation--rather than walks--as her primary mode of transportation. Bodies showing up on the mat today are simply quite different than the ones receiving asana instruction 50 to 100 years ago.

Consider also that, in the last 100 years, every major form of exercise and movement has evolved its training techniques. From running to gymnastics to cycling to dance to bodybuilding, every movement trains differently than it did just a few decades ago, due primarily to more advanced understandings of how bodies work.

When we put all these pieces together, it's undeniably bizarre that yogis insist on clinging to asana cues that are many decades old and outdated.

How do we relate this to body image?

Body image is the sum total of the thoughts, feelings, and associations we have about our bodies; it also refers to the value judgements we place on how our bodies look. Those value judgments stem from ideals and how we perceive ourselves to measure up to those ideals.

When yoga teachers teach or even suggest that a pose has a "correct" or "ideal" shape, we set students up for failure. Not every human body will fit into that ideal shape. This has the inevitable potential to make a student feel inadequate. For teachers to ignore or gloss over this fact--or to suggest that students must simply practice "yogic acceptance" when they don't meet these arbitrary ideals--is inconsiderate at best and negligent and dangerous at worst. When we do so, we abandon students who have a real and meetable need. Why should they have to suck it up and accept they can't meet our definition of the perfect asana when we could far more easily alter our language to provide a more realistic and anatomy-informed scope of alignment?

It's not an simple thing to ask. "Square your hips forward" and "drop your back foot 45 degrees" are easy to say. Anatomy-informed, body-positive cuing is harder. It takes more words and more on-the-fly thinking to respond to the needs of the bodies in the room. In Warrior 1, we might say, "Drop your back heel naturally in toward the midline of your mat. Allow your hips to open at a slight, natural angle as you square your shoulders forward." It's a lot more words. It's less rote and requires more work on the teacher's part.

And, perhaps hardest of all, it requires teachers to trust their students to feel what's best for their own bodies. Intimidating stuff for both the teacher (who may feel they're supposed to be "in control" of the class) and the student (who may have come to class expecting to just be told what to do).

Alignment's relationship to body image is simple: Body image arises in part from messages we get about our bodies, and yoga teachers must take care not to reinforce negative or limiting stereotypes about asana or students' bodies. Moreover, we must be mindful to send empowering, accepting messages through our cuing and not give in to lazy, old-fashioned language about poses.

I get it. Yogis get really tied to tradition. But it's important to remember that we have access to research and technology that our forebears could only dream of. I like to think that our wise, old gurus would have jumped at the chance to learn more about bodies and adjust their teaching accordingly.

And I think they'd approve of us doing the same.

CHAPTER 9
WHY I DON'T PRACTICE ASHTANGA

Ashtanga Yoga is revered in the West, and with good reason. It was one of the first styles of yoga brought to North America and gained a huge following in the middle-to-late part of the 20th century. It birthed many of the styles of Vinyasa Yoga practiced today. Pattabhi Jois--the father of Ashtanga yoga--is one of the most influential yoga teachers in modern memory.

I, too, respect the Ashtanga tradition. I get why people love it for its structure and discipline. I understand how and why it changes people's lives. I've sweated my way through led Primary Series classes and shown up for early morning Mysore practices. To use a tired cliche', some of my best friends are Ashtangis.

And yet, the longer I practice and teach, and the more I learn about the science of anatomy, the more I think Ashtanga gets it wrong and--in some cases--may be doing more harm than good. Here's why:

Those great teachers weren't anatomists. The Ashtanga lineage traces its roots back through Sri K. Pattabhi Jois to Sri T. Krishnamacharya. It's impossible to overstate the influence these men had on the practice of yoga in the 20th century. Both together and separately, they developed and codified a system of yoga that has been delivered to millions of people. But these men were not anatomy experts. While they were both learned men, neither had any formal education on the physical workings of the body. Because of this, their systems of yoga have some anatomical blind spots.

We know better now. In the last 30 years, scientific knowledge about the body has grown exponentially. We have new tools and techniques to help the body develop strength, flexibility, and overall health. Many styles of yoga have integrated this new information and evolved the practice in exciting and beneficial ways. I believe the role of yoga teachers is to grow the practice as new information becomes available, throwing out old and ineffective ways of moving in favor of new movement paradigms.

It's stuck in the past. Ashtanga yoga is taught very much the same way it was 50 years ago. No other movement discipline can say the same. Every type of movement--from running to dance to martial arts to elite-level sports--trains its practitioners very differently than it did half a century ago. This is precisely because of the gains in anatomical knowledge made in recent decades. Ashtanga yoga practitioners have steadfastly ignored anatomy research in favor of adherence to "tradition," leaving practitioners set up for injury and ineffective movement techniques.

Joints are treated badly. One of the most important outcomes of anatomy research in recent decades is a new understanding of what constitutes healthy movement. Simply put, healthy movement can be defined as "a little bit of movement from a lot of places." In other words, many joints and muscles must help make an action happen. The traditional cues of Ashtanga Yoga ask practitioners to do the opposite and force a lot of movement into a small number of places. For example, in any forward fold, Ashtangis are cued to "keep the spine straight and hinge at the hips." In other words, a lot of movement from a few places. This can put a great deal of compression on the hips and strain the lumbar vertebrae. Cues like this encourage unhealthy and injurious joint movement.

Muscles are treated badly. Muscles are designed to do certain jobs. It is possible, however, to train muscles to not do their job, which sets the body up for injury. For example, Ashtangis are taught to "relax the glutes" in backbends, with the erroneous assumption that doing so will allow for a deeper backbend. One of the functions of the glute muscles is to stabilize the sacrum and lumbar spine. When those muscles are trained to relax over time, the curvature of the backbend is shoved into the SI joints and lumbar vertebrae, creating an uneven and dangerous distribution of force in the joints. Moreover, as glutes and their surrounding muscles are trained to go slack when they should be working, the attachments of those muscles start to weaken. A common injury amongst advanced Ashtanga practitioners is a tearing of deep hip and gluteal joints away from the bones. (Yoga teacher Diane Bruni has written and spoken widely about her experience with this type of injury after many years of advanced Ashtanga practice. Her story is worth Googling.) This type of injury is intensely painful, takes a very long time to heal, and can be traced directly back to common cues of the Ashtanga practice.

Repetitive stress is real. I can't say this one enough: Repetitive stress is real. Doing the exact same motion over and over can and will injure your body. Ashtangis often practice the same series six days a week for years at a time. There are 60 Chaturangas in the Ashtanga Primary Series. Multiply that by six, and you have 360 Chaturangas a week. That's over 1400 Chaturangas a month. There's nothing inherently wrong with Chaturanga when performed with proper alignment, but that many per month for months or years at a time puts enormous strain on the shoulder girdle, rotator cuffs, wrists, elbows, and shoulder joints. Joints need a variety of movement over time to maintain health. Doing the same thing over and over puts unnecessary strain on joints and creates the potential for injury.

Deep adjustments are invasive and injurious... and they don't do what you think. A hallmark of the Ashtanga practice is deep adjustments applied by the teacher to get the student into the preferred alignment of the pose. Some Ashtanga teachers are sensitive enough to ask before touching a student, but many are not. It's impossible to know whether a student has experienced trauma or has some other reason to not wish to be touched. To lay hands on a student and manipulate them into poses their bodies might not be ready for could leave them feeling violated with no outlet to express that to the teacher. In addition, this type of manual manipulation puts the focus on what the teacher can do for the student, rather than what the student can do, thus disempowering the student and creating dependence on the teacher. And of course, manipulating someone's body into a space it's not ready to go on its own creates the potential for teacher-caused injury.

Bodies are more diverse than that. Human bodies come in a variety of shapes, sizes, and configurations. Some bodies have more adipose tissue to work with. Others have more longer bony protrusions in the skeleton, which means they hit bony compression in the joints sooner than others, limiting range of motion. Others have proportions that don't allow them to create certain shapes. Some bodies need to work on building flexibility; others need to develop strength. Ashtanga Yoga takes a one-size-fits-all approach to the human body that is simply unrealistic given the diversity of bodies that show up to the mat.

There is no perfect alignment. One of my teachers, Yoga Anatomy expert Leslie Kaminoff, says "Poses don't have alignment; people do." Ashtanga Yoga assumes that every body is capable of achieving every pose. Moreover, the system assumes that, if the practitioner cannot achieve a certain pose, it is the fault of the practitioner, not the pose. The traditional Ashtanga Yoga system ignores the inherent biodiversity of the human body in favor of false ideas about "perfect" alignment. In traditional Ashtanga Mysore rooms, a practitioner is often "tapped out" by the teacher if they can't achieve a pose, meaning they have to stop their practice at that point in the series, do the finishing series, and leave the room. This continues until the yogi achieves the pose, when they are granted permission by the teacher to move forward. This approach disempowers the student, shifting the focus from an intuitive relationship with the body to the teacher's assessment of a student's progress.

I want my practice to support my life. The more I study anatomy and student-teacher dynamics, the more I think Ashtanga often gets it wrong on an empirical level. But ultimately, practice is a subjective personal choice, and Ashtanga Yoga doesn't support the kind of life I want to live. I want a practice that builds self-compassion, not one that pushes me to "achieve" a pose. I want a practice that leaves me feeling empowered and intuitive, not one that forces me to depend on a teacher. And I want a practice that meets my needs in the moment, not a prescriptive series that doesn't take my unique needs into account.

Do I think people should stop practicing Ashtanga Yoga? Of course not. But I think it's important for yogis to question techniques that haven't evolved in decades. We can and must evolve our practices based on new anatomy research, and perhaps make the practices we love even better.

CHAPTER 10

WHAT WE NEED WHEN

I don't know her, but I do. Her mat is just inches from mine. She's young and fit and beautiful and very capable in her practice.

We sweat our way through the class next to each other.

She pushes herself hard. She flies through every vinyasa. She always takes the next, more advanced variation of the pose on offer. She moves quickly in her transitions and adds in extra movements and push-ups. She breathes hard and fast, always working for the next thing.

I recognize her.

She's me ten years ago.

I don't judge her. I know that feeling, that need to push on the mat. The need for the practice to be bigger and bolder with every breath.

For me, that hunt was about out-running my anxieties and insecurities. I confused exhaustion with relaxation. I walked out of classes sweaty and spent, and for a little while after, I didn't think about depression or anxiety or body image or any of the day-to-day stresses that plagued me.

I also felt like I had something to prove. I was young and fit and bendy, and I wanted my practice to show that I was capable on my mat. I wanted to be a "good" yogi with an "advanced" practice. My ego needed the validation of hearing the teacher say, "That's beautiful, Melissa!"

And I needed to feel the soreness the next day. I needed proof in my body that I had done something. I needed that lingering reminder that I was still a good yogi. I wore soreness like a badge of honor and proclaimed it, hoping that someone would ask me what I'd done to feel so achy.

I don't assume that the girl next to me on the mat that day was motivated by the same things that I was all those years ago. Maybe she just loves her practice. But her movements, her extra push-ups, her pushing to the next variation remind me so much of myself in my early and mid-20s. They reflect back to me how different my relationship with the poses is now.

My practice has softened so much over time. I still practice "strong" by most standards, but I move more slowly, and I'm not afraid to rest. I don't always push to the next, biggest variation, even if I know I could do it. Sometimes I bring my hands to my heart in Chair or Warrior 1, rather than extending them overhead, because that makes my shoulders feel happier. I used to feel self-conscious about doing those things in class, or not practicing as "strong" as I knew I could, because I was afraid of people judging me and having expectations because I'm a teacher. But after many years and many hours on my mat, my practice is fully mine, and I don't have anything to prove to anybody about it.

I used to practice "strong" because it was what I needed back then. I practice the way that I do because it's what I need right now.

I first published a version of the previous essay on the inherent alignment problems in Ashtanga yoga on a national website. I expected disagreement and was ready for some substantive debate. What I didn't expect was for people to take the post so personally. Members of my own yoga community reacted as if I was personally criticizing them for practicing Ashtanga, which was not at all my intention. Some comments became personal, criticizing both me and my teacher.

I was shocked by how vitriolic the conversation became. I come from an academic background where substantive critiques are not only welcomed, but considered necessary for the advancement of knowledge. For some reason, I'd pictured yogis thoughtfully nodding their heads and saying, "While I understand your points, if you examine the anatomical research of Dr. Guru Smith, you'll see…" I thought we'd compare notes and share knowledge and agree to disagree.

What I experienced instead was a reflection of the deeply personal nature of the practice. Yogis feel their practices intensely. They identify with them. Practice is a reflection of who we are in this moment.

The thing is, I totally understand the appeal of Ashtanga. I understand that people love it for its structure and discipline. I understand and honor that some yogis need to feel connected to a tradition. I understand that Ashtanga gives a sense of "progress" on the mat that few other styles can match. I understand how the ritual of a sequence can give birth to deep spiritual connection.

I recognize and honor that Ashtanga might give people exactly what they need at a certain time in their lives, and I would never want to denigrate that or take anything away from those dedicated practitioners. I know that they're getting what they need right now, and that, like me, their needs will likely change over time, and they might choose to explore other flavors and nuances in their practice.

Or not. And that's okay, too.

What shocked my most about the reaction to my Ashtanga essay was that people took my opinion so seriously. It was as if they felt I was trying to take their practice away from them. I said to several commenters, "I hope I don't have the power to to make you change what you do. I don't want that much responsibility!" I'm not the Yoga Police. I'm just one girl with an opinion who's logged a lot of hours on the mat.

My own practice is still evolving. Maybe it will soften more in the future. Maybe I'll need the strong, fast vinyasa I loved years ago. Maybe I'll even crave the structure and discipline of Ashtanga. But if there's one thing the practice has taught me, it's that I need to do exactly what's right for me, right now.

CHAPTER 11

SOMETIMES I NEED IT, TOO

I step back to my first Down Dog. My foot slips in a wet spot on my mat. It's too early in class for it to be sweat. Did I spill some water? Are the pipes in the ceiling leaking again? Why is my mat wet?

Oh yeah, I remember. It's tears.

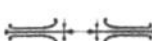

As a yoga teacher, I give a lot to a lot of people. I teach dozens of students a week. I hold space for them to sweat and feel and work on things. Sometimes people laugh; sometimes they get emotional. I support people in their process. I give people permission to cry, and I massage their heads in Savasana while they do. I love what I do, and I'm grateful for it.

On occasion, all this holding space for others convinces me that I have to be strong all the time, that it's not okay for me to be vulnerable, too. I rarely take classes, but when I do, stuff comes up for me, just like everyone else. I often feel like I have to hide in those moments and wait till I'm alone to process my stuff. I have to be the put-together teacher. I convince myself that I have to be okay so that my students will respect me.

But of course, this is false. It's my ego convincing me that I'm special and different, that the rules of humanity don't apply to me. I have just as many feelings and tough moments and insecurities as everyone else. And I have a right to come to my mat--whether in public or private--to work through those things.

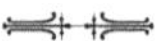

I'm not sure what moved me to take class that day, other than perhaps a desperate need to get out of the house and look at other human beings for an hour. I was exhausted from not sleeping and overthinking. I felt tears well up on the drive and almost turned around, but I made it to the studio, ragged and needy.

And of course--OF COURSE--the first pose was a restorative heart-opener. And OF COURSE the theme was vulnerability as a path to courage. And of course, I broke down and cried right there on my back, turning my face to the wall so no one would see me as tears rolled silently down my left cheek onto the mat.

It was an alignment-based class, taught by a friend who I think is a damn genius teacher. There was a lot of very focused shoulder work, the careful lifting of blocks and pulling mindfully against straps. At first, I didn't want all that energy near my heart; I felt like my chest was going to crack open if I had any more sensation there. But my friend kept me focused and in my body. She even made me laugh a little. Over time, the sensation dissipated and became easier to bear.

The class built to handstands at the wall. Much to my surprise, I felt strong when I kicked up, hovering in space for a few breaths, landing gently and with control. The focus on alignment felt grounding and focusing. I felt free to play, comforted to realize I could support my own weight. My teacher-friend held the space beautifully, maintaining the kind of compassionate control over a room that lets students relax and be led.

That's what we all need sometimes, to just relax and be led. To relinquish that needy, ego-fueled control over life and experience the moment.

I thought I would cry again in Savasana, but I didn't. I felt sad, but it was a tolerable sadness. My shoulders felt stabilized and integrated, as if they were able to once again hold up the weight of emotion.

I did cry again in the car on the way home. I'm human. Crying serves an important purpose, and thanks to my friend's class, I was able to embrace the tears rather than fight them. Yoga didn't solve all my problems that day, but it certainly made them easier to bear.

This lesson comes up for me over and over again. It's okay to teach, to lead, to stand in front of the class and be strong. It's also okay--and even more necessary--to take the student mat, let down some defenses, and allow myself to be led.

CHAPTER 12

HOW I PRACTICE NOW

When I first started practicing years ago, I had no idea what I was doing. I had a vague sense that poses should be in some type of order, but that order was a mystery to me. So I spent my time on the mat playfully stabbing at poses, holding them for 5 or 15 or 25 breaths. Warrior 2 on both sides, a wobbly Eagle for a minute, Tree Pose, a random Sun Salutation, some forward folds because I liked to stretch. It was unstructured and intuitive, as if I was introducing myself to the poses as much I was the poses to my body. "Hi, I'm Melissa. Can we be friends?" It was a wonderfully curious and investigative time in my life.

Later, I learned a bit more about sequencing and found some flow classes. I learned that poses can be linked together. I experimented with flow--Warrior 1 to Warrior 2 to Triangle. Sometimes I'd create a single, simple flow and do it over and over until I was tired. There was still very little method to my practice, but it didn't matter. My time on the mat was sacred and private. It freed me up to explore.

Years later, I'm grateful for those early, unstructured practices. Many yogis struggle for years to develop a home practice; I had one from the very beginning. I've never been attached to a teacher or a class. I've always been confident in my ability to do yoga on my own.

My practice has changed a great deal over the years. It has more structure now. I understand how to warm up, when to strengthen, when to stretch, how to capitalize on building heat, and when to cool down and rest. Where I used to dabble and experiment, my practice today is exclusively Core Strength Vinyasa now. Bent joints, wave-like movement, and a focus on Deep Core anatomy all feel like home to me on the mat. After almost 15 years of regular practice, I find that it's still constantly evolving, and I evolve within it.

My body bends easily. My muscles and fascia are naturally loose, and years of dance training in my youth trained them to stay pliable. I fall easily into splits and hip openers; my leg lifts effortlessly in Bird of Paradise. Flexibility has never been an issue. Strength is my struggle. Unlike some yogis, my muscles don't knot up easily into little balls of potential energy; they remain soft and mobile. Poses that require strength escape me. So I practice them. Over and over, I take on my own body weight and seek steadier balance, a longer hold. My body may never knot up with lean muscles, but I've learned to embrace the process of re-defining what strength means for me.

While I still work to get stronger, I no longer chase accomplishments on my mat. I see yogis on Instagram making bigger and more impressive asana shapes every day. There was a time when I would have jumped on that train and strained my body to keep up with social media yoga stars. As much fun as asana "challenges" and creating new shapes is, that kind of intensity no longer serves me. Life is intense enough. I need my practice to ground me, not shake me up.

Almost 15 years in, I recognize that my practice must support my life. It has to keep me strong enough to do what I need to do and feel good and flexible and healthy. But it can't dominate my life, nor can it leave me too exhausted and sore to do other things I love. Some yogis rise before dawn to practice for two hours or more. I'm not that kind of yogi, and I'm fine with that. My practice is a mid-day pause to re-center, a time when my mind is tired of work and my body craves movement.

And of course, at the center of every practice is compassion. It took a lot of years to learn to love this body of mine; many of those years I beat up on it pretty hard. But now I have and continue to practice compassion for this miracle of a body I get to walk around in. I love my loose and flexible muscles that may never feel totally comfortable in a handstand. I love my soft belly that houses incredibly strong core muscles. I love my arms that will never look toned, no matter how much muscle I build, but can hold a Crow pose for hours. I love my sweat and breath and the thousands of hours I've put in on my mat to bring me to this point in life. And I love knowing that my practice will be there for me, day after day, no matter what life throws my way next.

All these years and hours and breaths later, I sometimes still feel like that college girl who was just discovering yoga. Playfully stabbing at poses, curious about what it all means, and open to the deep mysteries to be uncovered--one breath at a time.

PART TWO:

Social Issues

CHAPTER 1

YOGA IN THE SOCIAL MEDIA AGE

I'm so grateful I started practicing yoga before social media became the ubiquitous beast it is today. When I first came to the mat in 2003, Yoga Journal magazine and DVDs were about the only places to find yoga outside of studios. Facebook was in its infancy and largely text-based, and one rarely experienced a deluge of images of hyper-advanced practitioners in contortionistic poses.

Today, yoga is practically the first thing you see on any social media app you pull up. There's no end to the pictures and videos of people in spandex doing impressive asana. Instagram "challenges" encourage home practitioners to play along and try new things on their mats. Yoga has had "celebrity" teachers for decades, but social media has given rise to a new breed of famous yogis, some of whom land book deals, DVD contracts, and tv appearances based solely on their online popularity.

I feel conflicted about the way yoga is portrayed in social media. In one sense, I love that social media has brought yoga to the masses and the masses to yoga. Instagram, Facebook, and YouTube provide access to yoga for free. People get to see a wide variety of yoga poses and styles without having to go to a studio or gym, which can be exclusive and cost-prohibitive. They can follow along at home without the pressure of feeling watched, eliminating the self-consciousness barrier that keep many people from trying yoga in a class setting. This also allows practitioners to develop a home practice, which is a struggle for many who get attached to studio practice and don't know how to move their bodies outside of a group class. In many ways, social media can take credit for yoga's ever-increasing popularity in the West.

However, much of what I see on social media makes me anxious. The posts that get the most views are the ones that are most impressive, which is to say that they're the least accessible to the majority of human bodies. I understand why that is: It's fascinating to look at a picture of a hyper-mobile, hyper-strong yogini balancing on one hand with both feet behind her head. But these pictures create an unrealistic expectation about what a yoga practice looks like and, worse, the possibility of comparison and the viewer feeling like they'll never be a "good enough" yogi. As the social media landscape becomes increasingly video-focused, transitions and flows become wilder and more choreographed, with more yogis trying the outrageous sequences they see on the internet without the guidance of a knowledgeable teacher.

The problem is that yoga--actual practice--isn't about a "wow" factor. Big poses are fun and inspiring, and a complex sequence can be exhilarating, but actual yoga practice is about dedication over time. A slower, less visually-impressive practice can be just as "deep" as a big, exciting one--and, depending on the practitioner, in many cases much deeper. But social media yoga can give the false impression that every practitioner should aim to do advanced poses.

Social media yoga also doesn't take into account the vast diversity of bodies in the world. Most of the yogis who achieve "celebrity" status on social media tend to have the same type of body: thin, naturally strong, and very flexible. This makes strong poses like Handstand or more contortionistic arm balances accessible, thus creating a multitude of opportunities for pretty pictures. Some body types simply don't have access to those types of poses; larger bodies, for example, might have extra tissue that prevents certain movements, while other body types hit bony compression in the joints that locks the yogi out of taking a particular shape. It's a simple fact: Diversity of anatomy doesn't allow all bodies to do the same things as all other bodies. Our diversity is part of what makes humans beautiful. However, diverse body types aren't always represented in yoga on social media.

This is the double-edged sword of yoga on social media: getting yoga to the masses on one hand while reinforcing exclusionary stereotypes on another. Yoga has always fought an uphill public relations battle in making the case that it actually is for everyone, not just lithe, young, bendy people. As yoga becomes increasingly visible on social media platforms, so too does the myth that only certain people can do yoga.

Perhaps even more insidious is how alarmingly White, cisgendered, and able-bodied the world of yoga celebrity is on social media. One struggles to find any representations of diversity at all amongst the most popular accounts. Given yoga's ability to help practitioners find union and wholeness both within and between groups, it seems that yogis should be more proactive about expanding the diversity of visual offerings in media, in hopes that all potential practitioners might see themselves represented on the mat and feel welcomed.

The unique thing about social media is its ability to be both self-aware and self-correcting. In the last couple of years, users have begun to call out the lack of diversity in visual representations of yoga, and counter-movements have sprung up. Social media is home base for the bod-positive movement, which asserts that all bodies are good bodies, regardless of size, shape, gender identity or expression, ability/disability, or any other factor. Body positivity has found a natural fit in the visual expression of asana, and more diverse users have stepped into the role of yoga influencers on social media. Larger-bodied yogis such as Amber Karnes, Jessamyn Stanley, and Dianne Bondy--the latter two being women of color--share their practices with thousands of followers every day. Instagram challenges encouraging yogis to share their limitations on the mat, as opposed to their "best" poses, pop up a few times a year.

Social media is far from done balancing the scales between white, fit, heteronormative practitioners and more diverse representations of what a yogi can look like. One struggles to find yogis with disabilities or those who are transgender, and the accounts that do exist lack the number of followers of more "traditional" social media yoga stars. There is still more work to be done to present an inclusive picture of the myriad ways to be a yogi, and the solution to the problem of underrepresented bodies on social media can only come from within social media itself.

This is our call, in this new era of yoga practice in an online world: We must show the reality of yoga. As a white woman with a moderately "advanced" practice and a body considered fit and able by most definitions, I certainly can't lead the charge on increasing diversity, but I can share the realities of my practice, such as poses I struggle with and ways I'm limited on my mat, to show that neither I nor my asana are perfect all the time. And I can most certainly encourage other yogis I know to share their diverse representations of yoga on social media.

The next step in making sure social media continues to recognize diverse practitioners is to continue to acknowledge the problem of white, fit, advanced yogis taking up most of the room in visual spaces and to actively work to highlight more diversity in those same spheres. All practices deserve to be celebrated, both in person and online, and it is we--everyday yogis with everyday practices--who must lead the charge in making sure that happens.

CHAPTER 2

BECAUSE I'M NOT THERE

Trigger Warning: Eating Disorders, Body Image

I vividly remember the first time I heard the term "thigh gap." I worked as a therapist at an eating disorder treatment center for about a year and a half, and the term came up during the weekly body image group I led. The clients, most of them 10 to 15 years younger than me, threw the term around casually, and I felt the weight of my age as I had to stop the conversation and ask what the term meant.

Although I'd never heard that particular term, a familiar ickiness washed over me as they explained the concept: "toes together, legs apart," meaning that your thighs don't touch each other, no matter how close you bring your feet. Ugh, I thought. Same old crap. You're only good enough when there's less of you.

The term thigh gap didn't exist when I was in the throes of my eating disorder in the late 90s and early 2000s, but the idealization of smallness certainly did. I came of age during the Kate Moss era, when collarbones, hip bones, and bones in general we in fashion. It is desirability defined by emptiness. Beauty defined by absence. It is the fetishizing of hollow cheeks and gaps between arms and ribs.

57

It is the belief that I'm only beautiful if I'm not there.

The thigh gap is only the latest iteration of this idea. Along with it came the "A4 challenge," a social media hashtag movement to demonstrate that one's waist disappears behind a piece of 8.5x11 paper (also called A4 paper), showing off one's thinness. It's abjectly terrifying to me that young women aspire to literally disappear behind a piece of paper as a mark of beauty and pride. But challenges like these are only the latest manifestation of a phenomenon that has oppressed women for centuries.

Female absence has often been rewarded throughout history. In some periods, a literal absence was required, with women expected to leave the room for "men's talk" and to not participate in discussions of politics and other matters of importance. In other eras, women could be present, but were expected to stay quiet and only speak when spoken to. Even today, the idea persists that women are expected to be dainty, demure, and quiet. Words like "ladylike" are still used to emphasize the constraints on women's behavior.

As women gained more power in the public sphere in the 20th century, female thinness was increasingly emphasized in beauty standards. This was especially evident in the 1960s--when a generation of women revolted, and subsequently Twiggy became the gold standard for beauty--and then again during the 1990s--when news outlets declared "The Year of the Woman," and heroin chic became the beauty rage soon after. This power and thinness seesaw cycles generationally. As soon as women gain some power in the public sphere, societal forces conspire to make sure they starve themselves. It's hard to revolt when you're frail and hungry. (This is not to denigrate women who are naturally thin. Many women are perfectly healthy in a thinner frame. My aim here is to highlight the fixation on artificial and unhealthy thinness for body types not designed to be so small, and the extreme measures required to create that thinness.) As women grow larger in presence, there's more pressure to be physically smaller. Society invents new places on a woman's body where there should be gaps and space. It's a manipulative mindfuck: See right here, where your body occupies a few square inches of space? That's wrong. You should vanish in just this area. Be absent right where I tell you to be.

Along with this absence comes the expectation of exaggerated presence in the areas where society deems it socially acceptable. Breasts should be large and full, and as "booty" culture gained mainstream popularity in the late 90s and beyond, backsides should be big and round. One might be tempted to celebrate the return of "curves" to female beauty standards, however, the only body parts that are allowed to be voluptuous are those that have been fetishized and hyper-sexualized for a heterosexual male gaze, emphasizing the fact that women are only allowed to "show up" if they're playing the role of a heteronormative sex object.

If breasts and booties are expected to be big and everything else must be small, how do women achieve the socially desirable hourglass shape? One alarming possibility surfaced in recent years, garnering social media attention and celebrity endorsements: waist trainers. Waist trainers are structured garments that fit around the midsection, holding it in tight. They're designed to be worn to the gym and during exercise, theoretically "training" the waist to get smaller. Women online report wearing their waist trainers for up to 16 hours a day in hopes of earning smaller and smaller waists. That's right: In the second decade of the 21st century--almost a century after women won the right to vote and 50 years after a generation of feminists fought for birth control and abortion rights--we've gone back to corsets, those barbaric antebellum devices that shrunk women down to 18-inch waists in hopes of finding a plantation-owning husband. Except now, women are expected to work out in them. Miss Scarlet, can you point me to my fainting couch?

As much as I rebel against the pervasive, oppressive restraints on women's physical forms, part of my brain still buys into them. I gained a little weight last year, and it freaked me out. I stressed and cried about it, just like I did when I was an eating-disorder-afflict-ed teenager. I lamented that I wasn't as "pretty" as I had been just a year before. But as I approached the ten-year anniversary of my eating disorder recovery, the wiser part of my brain and heart took over, reminding me of hard-earned lessons from years of therapy, yoga, and personal growth work: I am not my body. I am a strong, successful woman. I have a good life. I am beautiful just the way I am. And after a lot of life and lessons and overcoming challenges, I believe I've earned the right to take up a little more space on this planet.

And perhaps that should be a benchmark in the fight against sexism and misogynistic oppression: When women are allowed to occupy any body, no matter how spacious, we will know our value is recognized. We are not beautiful in our absence, but in our presence, and the more space we claim, the louder we speak, and bigger and bolder we live our lives, the more we share our intrinsic, divine beauty with the world.

CHAPTER 3

WHY I TALK ABOUT BODY IMAGE

Trigger Warning: Body Image

"I'm not really clear on what you're doing here. You're just posting pictures of yourself doing yoga with no shirt on?"

"All I see is a woman with a great body showing off yoga poses and claiming it has something to do with body image."

"What do you have to worry about? Leave the body image talk to people who actually struggle with their bodies."

When I started my hashtag #noshirtnoshoesnoshame--which encourages yogis of all shapes and sizes to bare their bellies in yoga poses to promote body acceptance--I was nervous. I made the conscious choice to expose my body in a way I never had before. For the most part, I received positive and supportive comments. But--unsurprisingly, given the inherent negativity found in online comments sections--I also heard a small but persistent chorus of people asking, "What do you have to worry about?"

I get it. I'm a "skinny" girl. (Sort of. More about that later.) I have a handful of toned muscles and can fill out a pair of jeans pretty well. Most people would look at me and say that I'm close in size to the cultural ideal. I look fit and healthy and, by most measures, attractive.

And I still struggle with body image. And, despite comment sections that might want me to keep my mouth shut, I'm going to talk about it.

I'm going to talk about it because it's my truth; I fought hard to overcome a decade-long eating disorder, and fighting lingering body image issues is how I choose to stay healthy. I'm going to talk about it because it's a feminist issue; body image struggles are a reflection of how women are represented in the media and treated in public spaces. And I'm going to talk about it because I want to create safe spaces where other women--of all shapes, sizes, and backgrounds--can talk about their struggles, too.

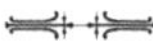

Let me pause here and recognize my own privilege. I fully acknowledge that I benefit from thin privilege. I can walk into almost any mainstream store in the country and find clothes in my size. I don't have to worry about fitting into seats in public venues or, worse yet, being shamed for needing a larger-sized chair. People are less likely to comment on the amount of food on my plate than my larger sisters (although that does happen sometimes). I also benefit from the "halo effect," in which people unconsciously assign positive character traits--such as intelligence, kindness, and work ethic--to others they perceive to be attractive.

In most brands, I'm size 4/6. I hover between a Small and a Medium, depending on where I shop. I'm pretty evenly proportioned. My stomach (historically my "problem" area) is relatively flat and even has a little muscle definition at this point in my life.

But my body is far from perfect. I have cellulite. Everywhere. My thighs, my butt, my upper arms. I tend toward softness, making tone hard to come by, even for this exercise junkie. My muscle mass builds up in loose bundles, which makes me look bulky and solid.

And I'm far from immune to body comments. As a yoga teacher, my body is very public. People often comment on my size or parts of my body or how I look in clothes. Even when these comments are intended as favorable, they still make me self-conscious and remind me that women can never get away from scrutiny. Members of my own yoga community have gone out of their way to comment when I've gained weight or to compare my size or shape to another yoga teacher. While I may have "nothing to worry about" according to some, others want to make sure that I do worry about whatever perceived imperfections I may have.

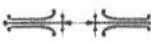

All women--no matter their size or shape--are told they aren't good enough. Thin women can never be thin enough… to a point. And then suddenly they're "too thin," "anorexic," and "disgusting". If you happen to hit the magical right size, then your boobs or your butt are too small. Or your skin tone isn't right. Or your nose is weird.

Or worse yet, you're told you "have nothing to worry about" and are shut out of the body image conversation all together.

This is the most damaging thing you can say to anyone trying to share their own story, regardless of the details. This renders the person sharing invisible. It minimizes and de-legitimizes a struggle that reflects very real, very persistent problems in society's relationship with women.

Let's stop telling women that they don't have a right to feel the way they feel.

Cultural body ideals are based on a variety of different opinions about what looks most attractive. Big butt, small butt, skinny, curves, muscles, no muscles. Because opinions vary widely, women end up ping-ponging between different representations of ideal and are left exhausted and discouraged, realizing that we'll never be good enough, no matter what we do. Not a single one of us are immune from cultural scrutiny and "not good enough" messages. We're all affected. All day, every day.

I talk about body image because, after years of struggle, I've recognized that I have the power to free myself from adherence to unrealistic cultural ideals. I have the power to define what is healthy and good enough for my perfectly imperfect body. I have the power to accept myself and witness the unique miracle of a physical form I get to travel around in.

I talk about body image because I want to create a world in which all women are considered good enough. And I want to bring my sisters with me.

CHAPTER 4

THE PRIVILEGE LETTERS

When I first learned about the concept of societal privilege, I had the same reaction a lot of people with privilege have: Nuh uh! I don't have any kind of special privileges! My life has been hard, and I've worked for everything I have. Lots of people have tried to hurt me, and I've overcome it all. Society hasn't given me anything special!

Oh, how much I had to learn.

And fortunately, I did learn, thanks to the patient mentorship of professors, mentors, and friends, who gently pointed out how oppression shows up in society until I was able to internalize it and begin to make changes in my own perceptions and behavior.

The truth is, I have immense privilege. I'm a straight, white, cisgender, upper-middle class, native English-speaking, able-bodied, thin person with with educated parents who myself holds not one but two post-secondary degrees. The mountain of privilege I stand on is so tall, it's a wonder there's still oxygen up here. Doors open for me every day that would not open for someone with different societal descriptors. Not a day goes by that I don't move through the world with ease. In many ways, my life is pretty sweet.

And yet, I've struggled. I've experienced many of the unique ways women are oppressed in Western society. I come from a challenging childhood background that left me with the scars of trauma and lifelong depression. I've battled an eating disorder and fought to overcome the trauma of rape. My life might be sweet, but it hasn't been easy.

And both of those things can be true at the same time.

The thing about acknowledging privilege is that it asks us to hold onto some paradoxes. You can have privilege and still struggle. You can have privilege and hurt. You can have privilege and still not be happy.

But you still have privilege.

It's only in recent years that I've really meditated on privilege and its consequences in my life and more broadly. The journey toward awareness presents many humbling challenges, mostly to my ego. But overall, I think that this awareness has set me on a path toward becoming a better, more compassionate person to the ways people around me are oppressed.

I wanted to write about privilege for this book, because I think it's such a massively important topic. But I'm no expert. I can't take an academic perspective on it yet, as I'm still learning.

Instead, I'd rather talk to people like me, people who experience privilege blindly every day and might feel defensive when the topic comes up. Some of the stuff I've been fortunate enough to learn is stuff we all need to hear.

And so, my friends, these letters are for you, from my heart, in hopes that the messages within might be as helpful for you as they have been for me.

⚍╬╬⚎

Dear White People,

We need to talk.

Y'all. We're the problem.

I know, I fought that thought for a long time, too. It's okay to acknowledge your resistance to it. It might even make you feel angry, and that's okay, too. But can you, just for a moment, take a deep breath, set those feelings aside, and be open to hearing me?

White people are historical oppressors. You know slavery? Yeah, that was us. (I recognize that there are historical examples of people of color enslaving others, but there's no doubt that the vast majority of enslavement was done by white people. And in the United States, enslavement of Black people by whites is the only relevant example.) Even though slavery was abolished in this country over 150 years ago, white people still oppress other races through legislation, workplace policies, and everyday behavior. We do dumb things like ask people of color to take our "feelings" into account while they're actively and systematically being oppressed. And then we do dumber things like deny that racism is still a problem in this country and sweep the lived experiences of people of color under the rug.

When we talk about things like "reverse discrimination," we totally invalidate the pain and fear people of color feel throughout their lifetime in overt and covert experiences of racism. Hear me say this: No white person will experience as much racial discrimination in their entire lifetime as a person of color experiences in a single month. This is a fact. It's been empirically proven. It's not up for discussion.

Are you "yes, but"-ing me right now?

Stop. Take a deep breath. Let me ask you some questions.

When you walk down the street as a white person, do people ever cross to the other side of the street to get away from you?

Do you routinely get followed around by security personnel in stores just because of the color of your skin?

Do you have to worry about yourself or members of your family getting shot by police officers when you or they have done nothing wrong?

People of color deal with this kind of stuff and much more every single day.

Are you saying "But I've dealt with…" right now?

Stop. Take a deep breath. Hear me say this.

Just because you have privilege in one area of your life doesn't mean you don't or won't face challenges. And your privilege doesn't invalidate any personal pain you've experienced in your life.

You can be white and still struggle. You can be white and experience pain. You can be white and have hardships in your life.

But to pretend for one second that you've experienced even a fraction of the discrimination that people of color experience on a daily basis is heartless and self-centered. And we have to get real about that.

I speak from a very small amount of experience here. Acknowledging my white privilege set me on a path toward being a better person. I'm a baby in this arena, but just having the veil pulled from in front of my eyes a little bit has made me more compassionate toward the people of color in my life. I'm more open in conversation and a better listener. And more importantly, I want to keep learning. I want to sit down and shut up and hear what people of color experience on a daily basis so that I can know how to effectively help. And not how I might want to help, but what people of color might want or need me to do to actually be effective.

Having white privilege doesn't make you a bad person. You didn't choose to have it. You were born how you were born, and you can't change it. But denying it doesn't make the problem any better. The very best thing you can do is acknowledge and accept, "Yes, I benefit from white privilege. That is a reality in my life."

Our whiteness can make us effective allies in the fight against racism when the time is right. Because we're white, many people (unfortunately) will listen to us first before they will listen to our brothers and sisters of color. We can be powerfully effective in some cases if we draw attention to racial issues, then yield the floor to people of color to share their personal stories and perspectives.

But we have to be willing to yield the floor.

We have to know when to shut up and let other people speak. This is hard for us, because, as white people, we're used to thinking people care about what we have to say. But sometimes--often, in fact--it's not about us.

Please, fellow white people, don't feel shame about your white privilege. And please don't give into anger when someone points it out to you. These feelings are blocks to anything ever actually getting better and will keep you stuck in unconscious cycles of oppressing those around you. Instead, take a deep breath, mindfully acknowledge your privilege, and commit to growing and learning how to use it for good.

If we're all willing to do that, we can look forward to being a part of the much needed solution.

Love,
A White Girl

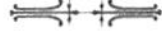

Dear Thin Yoga Teacher,

I see you.

Your Instagram posts are beautiful. You look so lithe and strong in your poses. I know you enjoy growing your practice, and the bigger the poses you can do, the more people see and like your posts. You are inspiring.

But sometimes, I get concerned about the things you post. You talk about cleanses and offer to post before and after photos. You're already so thin; what exactly are you hoping to see in the "after"? I worry that you think your body isn't good enough the way it is. I worry that you don't see yourself the way others see you.

I worry that you might be perpetuating the oppression of a phenomenon known as Thin Privilege.

I can hear right now my sisters who say, "But there's no such thing as thin privilege! I've been made fun of my whole life for being skinny. I've been called names. Guys made fun of my flat chest and skinny legs. Thin people are just a discriminated against as fat people."

First, I'm so sorry you dealt with bullying and verbal abuse. There's no excuse for cruelty.

Second, you can have privilege and still struggle. And just because you've struggled doesn't mean you don't have privilege.

I know this from my own journey. As a woman who's never been larger than a size 6, but who has also struggled with body image for as long as I remember, I've had to work hard to come to terms with the concept of thin privilege. How could this thing I've battled with for so long, that I woke up every morning despising, afford me any benefit in society?

But as I dove into the work of body positivity, I learned from my sisters with larger bodies just how prevalent fat-shaming and fat oppression are, perpetuated by the realities of thin privilege. The more I listened, the more I learned. And it this new awareness has changed the way I talk about my body in public. Rather than minimizing my body image struggles, it gave me a new context in which to see them, and empowered me to take steps to change the dialogue around women's bodies so that no one has to feel ashamed of how they look.

I believe it's so important that we acknowledge the ways in which we benefit from thin privilege. You and I, as women who are considered "fit" by society, are judged far less than our brothers and sisters in larger bodies. We are less likely to be thought of as stupid or lazy on first impression. We don't have to think about whether or not we'll fit in the seat at a theater or on an airplane. We don't have to worry about strangers commenting on how much we eat in public or giving us unsolicited health advice. We can walk into any typical store and find clothes in our size.

The sad reality is that thin people are treated as morally superior in our society. Studies have shown that we're viewed as more disciplined and healthier. We're considered smarter and more fun to be around. These facts of perception are born out in research over and over again.

If you add in conventionally accepted notions of attractiveness--such as smooth skin, bright eyes, and symmetrical features--we become the beneficiaries of the "halo effect," which means people unconsciously attribute positive character traits to us regardless of whether or not we actually possess them.

And none of this is our fault. We don't ask to be seen as morally superior to our brothers and sisters in larger bodies. Decades of media messaging and social convention have added up to create these widely accepted perceptions. Hyper-visual social media culture only compounds the detrimental effects of fat oppression and thin privilege.

As thin women, we suffer at the hands of thin privilege, as well. Even when we're thin, we're not thin enough. The slightest weight gain is cause for angst. We feel pressure to maintain our figures and conform to very tight standards of beauty.

All of this is exhausting. And it sucks.

I see this dynamic playing out in a supremely toxic way in our beloved yoga community. As yoga has been folded into the hyper-visual world of social media, our asana bodies are on full display, subject to criticism and critique, which can feel terribly vulnerable. Teachers are especially subject to this vulnerability, as we "brand" ourselves and use asana pictures to catch the attention of potential students. It's easy to believe that we, our bodies, and our poses must all be perfect to showcase our teaching skills.

Unfortunately, social media provides a space where yogic practices can be warped and weaponized in pursuit of this perfection. Cleanses--which are functionally crash diets--for example, take on spiritual overtones. The extreme calorie restriction of a cleanse somehow makes us morally superior, and if we post about it on social media, our students might feel inspired (pressured?) to follow suit.

Meanwhile, all we're doing is perpetuating the message that our bodies aren't good enough the way they are. And in the context of thin privilege and student-teacher power dynamics, this message can be incredibly damaging to our students' self-image.

As teachers, we have a responsibility to at least try to see ourselves as our students see us. They will put us on a pedestal in a heartbeat. We may not like this feeling, but we can't control it. Our students will look to us for how to behave and think about their bodies. If we cleanse, they will think they need to cleanse. If we focus on our perceived flaws and imperfections, they'll focus on theirs, as well.

And they'll compare themselves to us. If we, who are more flexible than the average person, post about how we need to be more flexible, how can they not think, "If she thinks she's not flexible enough, what must she think of me?"

And if we, who are perceived as thin and fit and healthy, post about needing to cleanse or imply that we need to lose weight, how can they help but think, "If she thinks she needs to lose weight, she must think I'm disgusting"?

And can we even imagine how triggering all of this body talk must be for someone struggling with an eating disorder?

As yoga teachers, we have great responsibility in how we present ourselves to the world. We can either be bastions of body positivity or we can perpetuate the same hurtful messages that oppress all women everywhere in regard to their bodies. I believe it's imperative that we set the example for body acceptance and self-love.

And most of all, I want you to know how beautiful you already are. You're perfect, just as we're all already perfect, regardless of our size, shape or ability. You don't need a cleanse or a pose to prove that to yourself or anyone else.

I hope that you'll pause and think before you make that next post. And, most of all I hope that, the next time you look in the mirror, you see your beauty, just like I do.

Love,
A Thin Yoga Teacher

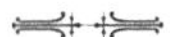

Dear straight, cisgender, educated, English-speaking, able-bodied people,

Y'all, we have to be more aware. We have to be more attentive in our language and our attitudes. There are people in the world who face discrimination the likes of which we can't fathom. We need to be more sensitive.

I'm tired of seeing the word "sensitive" vilified and mocked. I'm tired of words like "snowflake" to describe people who try to make the world a little better for people who have less privilege than others. What's wrong with being sensitive? My sensitivity makes me kinder and more accepting. Since when is that a bad thing?

We move through the world with such ease. We can walk into public spaces and easily communicate. Hell, we can physically walk in the door without having to look for the wheelchair ramp, which might be on the backside of the building. Our education means we aren't judged for how we speak or what we don't know. We don't have to worry about whether we'll be attacked for loving the person we love, even though our marriage is now legal in this country. We don't have to agonize over which bathroom we're allowed to use and whether we'll be safe when we walk in there.

The fact is that most of us stand on a mountain of privilege every day. We can't see it, because to us, it's just the ground beneath our feet, and the view around us is simply what we're used to from our vantage point. When confronted with the notion that we benefit from privilege, we have two choices: to deny it, or to acknowledge it and learn.

When we deny our privilege, we inevitably and unknowingly perpetuate the oppression privilege creates. To deny privilege is to assume that we came to our station in life through our own internal merits, which is only ever partially true. When we make those kinds of assumptions, we project them onto those who have less privilege than we do, which leads to stereotypes of minority groups being lazy or less capable--which lead to attitudes and behaviors that oppress those minority groups. The truth is, they're not lazy, they're simply fighting a much harder battle than we are, one that is invisible to us from where we stand.

When we choose to acknowledge our privilege and learn from it, however, we begin to break the cycle of oppression. We can start to see the perspective of those who fight oppression daily and, with increased knowledge and sensitivity, stand with them in that fight. We, in our privilege, can be powerful allies in the fight for equality.

Hear me say this: Acknowledging your privilege doesn't make you a bad person. You didn't choose it; you were born into it through a circumstantial lottery over which you had no control. Acknowledging privilege isn't easy. It requires humility and openness that can be hard to access. But ultimately, this learning process makes us better, kinder, more loving human beings.

Acknowledging your privilege will make you a better person. I promise.

And then, of course, comes the question: After acknowledging it, what do I do with it? Now what?

First and foremost, we must listen. People in positions of privilege are notoriously bad at listening to minority groups, preferring instead to speak, since we're used to being the ones who are listened to. To break the cycle of oppression, we must be willing to take a seat and listen. In listening, we will learn where and how we can be effective in helping down the road.

Second, we must watch our language. Oppression sneaks insidiously into the words we use, and so we must learn to be sensitive in our word choices. Hopefully we all know enough by now not to use words like "gay" and "retarded" to mean stupid, and if we don't, now is a good time to commit to not using those words anymore. Perhaps also pay attention to whether your language is gendered, sexist, and heteronormative. Do you automatically use the pronoun "he" when referring to doctors, or "she" when referring to teachers? Do you ask male acquaintances "Do you have a girlfriend?" rather than the gender-neutral equivalent, "Do you have a partner?" Do you assume what gender people identify with rather than asking the simple and respectful, "What pronouns do you use?" These language shifts are simple but powerful ways to communicate openness and willingness to not perpetuate cycles of oppression.

Finally, we must keep listening. Growing up in privilege leaves us with blind spots to others' experiences, and so, we must never grow weary of listening to the experiences of those who experience oppression to that we can learn and grow. Learning and growth must become our highest values as we commit to standing against oppression in all its many forms.

Indeed, we can and must make recognizing privilege a spiritual practice, as we strive for our own internal growth.

This work can be hard and scary, but simply showing up for it sets us on the path to change. Be humble, be aware, and be willing. In doing so, we help ourselves and the many others around us who need us to stand with them.

We're all in this together.

Love,
Melissa

CHAPTER 5

LET'S GET PISSED: A YOGI'S RESPONSE TO FERGUSON & OTHER POLICE SHOOTINGS

Trigger Warning: Violence, Racism

The shooting of Michael Brown in Ferguson, MO in 2014--and the subsequent exoneration of the police officer who shot him--affected me deeply. In fact, it was arguably the event that put concepts of white privilege and racial oppression squarely in my view, especially as they nascent Black Lives Matter movement gained momentum in the wake of multiple shootings of this kind. After this shooting in particular, I felt hopeless and angry that black people had to live in a different reality than I do.

As I talked about my feelings about the decision that exonerated the police officer who shot Michael Brown, as I lamented my feelings of helplessness and wondered out loud what more I could do, I was stunned into silence as someone in my yoga world told me, "You need to stay out of it. This isn't your fight."

I disagree. This is my fight. This is everyone's fight. And I want more yogis to be as angry about it as I am.

Yogis often run from anger. We regard it as dark and unenlightened. We avoid it because we think it is the opposite of the floating-on-the-clouds, lovey-dovey types we think we're supposed to be. This is a narrow view of anger. Anger can be fierce and righteous and motivating. Think of the goddess Kali. Think of Jesus in the temple, turning over tables. Anger has its place on the path to enlightenment. Anger points us to the places in which shadow can and must be turned to light.

I'm not angry about the decision in Ferguson because I know whether Michael Brown was or wasn't antagonizing the police officer. I wasn't there. I'm not angry because I know that he was a "good kid." I never met him. I'm not angry because I think the police officer was corrupt or poorly trained. I've never met him either.

I'm angry because Michael Brown's life was treated as unimportant, because the grand jury decided his death wasn't even worth looking into in the court of law. I'm angry because, as a yogi, I know that all lives are connected. I'm angry because the devaluing of Michael Brown's life might as well be the devaluing of my life and the lives of everyone I love.

Michael Brown was a human being, just like me. He had flaws (no more than I do, I assure you). He loved his family. He laughed about things he found funny. He probably worried about the future, just like we all do at some point. He had friends, a favorite color, and hopes and dreams. He felt all the things I've felt: joy, sadness, longing, anger, and fear.

If I am truly to believe the yogic teachings--the ones I espouse in my classes and workshops week after week--all beings are One. All beings are manifestations of the Divine, none greater or lesser than any other, and we are all interconnected on a deeper and higher level than we can fathom. To say that Michael Brown's death didn't deserve a day in court--to say that this one death is dismissible--is to say that all lives are meaningless. If one life can be treated so callously, no lives are sacred.

And that makes me angry.

Gandhi said, "I regard myself as a soldier of peace." Yogis, we must be foot soldiers in the fight for equality, which ultimately is the fight for the honoring of divinity of all beings. I'm not asking you to take to the streets or engage in acts of extremism. But we simply have to stop being so passive. Yogis are uniquely suited to recognize injustice. We are over 30 million strong in the United States alone, many of us well-educated and blessed with leisure time and disposable income. We have a strong and meaningful voice in this country, and it's time we begin to mobilize and use it.

As you watch the events like the ones in Ferguson unfold, do not sit and wring your hands and hide behind passivity in the same of being spiritual. Make a meditation of writing letters to the editor or to your lawmakers. Organize peaceful protests in the tradition of great spiritual leaders like Gandhi and Martin Luther King, Jr. Show up to rallies with the same intention and grace you do to your mat.

Let's be soldiers of peace. This is our fight, too.

CHAPTER 6

MAKING MEANING

Trigger Warning: Violence

On the afternoon of April 16th, 2007, I was sitting outside the Starbucks in Five Points, drinking a cup of coffee, eating a bag of sweet potato chips, and killing time before my grad school class that evening. When my phone rang, I wasn't terribly surprised to see it was my cousin Liz. She and I worked at a summer camp together which was starting in a few weeks, so I assumed she was calling to talk over some camp business.

When I answered, she said, "Have you heard about the shootings at Virginia Tech this morning?"

"Yes," I said. Everyone had. It had been all over the news all day.

"You know that's where Ryan Clark goes, right?" Ryan was a very dear mutual friend of ours from camp. He was our Music Director and had become like family to Liz and me, as well as many others.

"Ryan was shot this morning. And he did pass away."

I don't remember much about the next few minutes. Everything took on a surreal quality, like I was staring down at my life through a very long, thin tube. I know that I stood up in the middle of the crowded street, burst into tears, and screamed "Are you serious?!" into the phone. I know I took off running down the street, tears streaming from my face and sobs bursting from my chest, sprinting back to my car, unsure of where exactly I was going but knowing I needed to get somewhere, anywhere, away from this unfathomable reality. And I know for an absolute certainty that my world came to a jarring, screeching halt in that moment.

Why? The question rang like bells in my head for weeks. How? What purpose? Why him? Why now? Why such violence? Why? Why? Why? The question would wake me up at night. It would force me to walk out of class in tears, seeking solitude in the nearest public restroom. It would pull be out of line at the grocery store, because there was yet another magazine cover with his face on it, and I just couldn't be confronted with a face I would never see again, a smile I would never share again. Not here, not in public.

A national tragedy is a loss unlike any other. There's no room to mourn in private, like there usually is when a loved one passes away. This is News, and everyone wants to talk about it all the time for weeks. You can't turn on a radio or television without being reminded that the person you love is gone. You can't escape from thinking about it because, on a national scale, it's What We're All Thinking About Right Now. The person you love is no longer yours, but the nation's, a celebrity to be discussed and analyzed and speculated about. It doesn't matter that you knew them, because now the nation knows them, and that's what's most important.

But then, weeks later, when you're finally ready to talk about your own grief, your own unending, gut-wrenching sadness, everyone else has moved on to the next major news story. Your heartbreak is yesterday's news. And just when you need that support most, you're often left alone in your grief.

Any time a mass shooting like the one at Sandy Hook Elementary in Newtown, CT or Pulse Nightclub in Orlando, FL happens, my heart gets ripped out all over again. I remember those terrifying days of coming to terms with the finality of it all. I remember the burden of the constant media attention to what felt, for me, like such a personal moment. The shooting at Sandy Hook Elementary last Friday was especially hard because most of the losses were children. I lost a dear friend, which was tremendously hard, but I didn't lose a child. I can only imagine the magnitude of grief those families are feeling. Violent and senseless don't begin to cover it.

It is our nature as humans to, soon after a tragedy like this say, "Now what?" Where do we go from here? How to we make sense of the senseless and give some kind of meaning to the experience? Everyone chooses their own path. Some will choose to discuss gun laws, a meaningful and worthwhile debate. Others will focus on supporting the families and community directly affected. Still others will put energy into improving mental health services in hopes of preventing future events like this. And others will, for a while at least, shut down. They will run from the grief and feelings of powerlessness and go on about their lives hoping that if they pretend nothing happened, it might come true one day.

For many months after the Virginia Tech shootings, I was one of the latter. I told very few people about my profound loss. I avoided all media and sat quietly in my grief. I reached out only to my camp family, because they understood my pain. They felt it, too, exactly as I did, but many of them lived far away, and many of my hometown friends had no idea what I was feeling. It was a horribly lonely time.

Then one day, something shifted. Whether I got tired of feeling so alone or finally got strong enough and healed enough to do something different, I don't know. But I needed to do something. I needed for Ryan's death to not be in vain. I needed him to be more than a fading headline. I needed to honor his memory in some way.

So I chose to be more like him. The things that I admired most about Ryan were his compassion, his openness, his sense of humor, and his integrity. But above all else, I admired his authenticity. He was totally and completely himself. Genuine, unique, unafraid. I made a conscious decision to live more like Ryan had lived and to inspire others to do the same. A few months after his death, I enrolled in yoga teacher training, something I'd been wanted to do for a long time but had been too afraid to attempt. When the day came to choose the word that sums up our teaching approach, I shared with my fellow trainees about how Ryan's loss had affected me so deeply. In his honor, I chose as my word "authenticity." In every class I teach, I try to convey the message that it's okay to be completely yourself, because that's what Ryan taught me.

In the weeks and months after a mass shooting, we will all try to make sense of the horrendous events in our own ways. Like most people, I have no answers for why this continues to happen in our country and no words of wisdom. But as someone who's been directly touched by a national tragedy, I hope that you will continue to remember the victim's families and friends long after the headlines fade. They surely appreciate the public support in the short-term, but many may not be in a position to receive it. And they need support even more months after the event, after the camera crews leave and they must continue on with daily life without they ones they loved.

I also hope we can all find ways to honor the victims in our own lives. Honor Vicki Soto, the brave first-grade teacher at Sandy Hook who hid her students in closets and died protecting them, by standing up for what you believe in, no matter the cost. Honor grieving parents by paying special attention to the children in your life, making sure they know they're loved. Honor the victims of the Pulse Nightclub shooting by supporting LGBT causes in your own community.

While these obscene shootings are devastating and traumatic. They don't have to be in vain. We can turn our tragedies into moments of strength, and our pain into deeper opportunities for love.

CHAPTER 7

DIVISION & YOKING

"**N**O BAN... NO WALL! NO BAN... NO WALL!"
I'm standing in the Birmingham Airport with 3000 other protesters. We're holding signs that say things like "We're All Immigrants." Some signs make puns about the current administration, or quote sections of the Constitution. We shout slogans of support and unity. Impassioned speakers talk about togetherness and community. We stand together in opposition of the travel ban the White House announced the night before.

We are united... I think.

As I listen to the speakers from the Black Lives Matter movement, the local Hispanic community, and the local Muslim community, I look around. As I survey the crowd, I notice something striking: Everyone is standing with and talking to people of their own race. All around me, people are clumped together by racial and ethnic group. Whites talk to whites. Black people talk to one another. Hispanic and Muslim people stand in twos and threes.

A few feet to my right stand three Muslim women, identifiable by their headscarves, long sleeves, and floor-length skirts. They stand alone, silent. No one is speaking to them. Even as the mostly white crowd shouts slogan of support and unity, most people avoid eye contact with them. Their separateness is palpable.

Suddenly, I'm overcome with shame. I feel like a white dumb-ass.

This is the problem. This is why well-intentioned White people get made fun of, and with good reason. We'll wear our shirts and hold our signs and donate our money and post things on Facebook. But when it comes to actually doing something, like interacting with people of color during times of crisis, we often fail miserably.

I believe White people really do care. I know I do. We do the best we can to show our support. Unfortunately, we just don't have the insight into the experiences of people of color to innately know how to help. But we can learn. We can be effective in helping heal the division in our country.

Right now, we need to come together more than ever. Our country feels so divided, and people of color, LGBT citizens, and other marginalized groups are watching their rights stripped away by the current administration. White people (and straight and cisgendered people) have the opportunity to use their privilege to speak up against these injustices. It's great that we show up to marches and make our presence known. But what else can we actually do to address the problems of division in our country?

In wrestling with this problem, I turned to my yogic teachings for answers. Surely the ancient masters gave us some guidance in how to address painful divisions.

The word "yoga" comes from the Sanskrit root word yuj which translates roughly as "to yoke" or "to join together." Often this translation is applied to the uniting of breath and movement, or of body and mind, or of physical and spiritual. One of yoga's other super powers is its ability to bring people together. If you've ever been to a yoga festival, you know what I'm talking about. People love to get together on their mats to move and breathe in unison. Yes, most of these events are predominantly white, and that problem needs to be addressed by the yoga community. But from my experience, yoga has as much power as music to unite people in common purpose.

If yoga has taught me nothing else, it's that I must be strong in myself in order to connect with other people. My internal systems must be united and healthy in order to fully unite with others. If I try to connect with people when I'm not fully integrated--mind, body, and spirit--my ego will get in the way, and I'll try to make that interaction about me, or I won't be as fully loving and compassionate as I'd like to be. This gets in the way when I try to show up in support of people of color and other groups experiencing oppression. In those situations, I can't make it about me. I have to be able to focus my compassion and my efforts on the needs of others. I have to be willing to step back and let others speak, which I can only do if my ego is in check. I need to be able to take a step back, breathe, and willingly give to others.

As we face the division in our country at this time, I believe it's important that we focus first on our own internal divisions. In order to come together, we must first be united within. Our own pain and prejudices can't get in the way of our support for others. We must show up in those spaces as a whole self.

At the airport that day, the speakers wrapped up and the crowd began marching again. In a moment of wishing to do something, I approached the three Muslim women. I felt my own nerves jangling my body. I have no idea what to say beyond a desire to say something, anything, to them.

"Hi, I'm Melissa. Can I give you a hug?"

They smile politely and say yes. As I hug each of them in turn, I say, "We're with you. We support you." They are very sweet as they hug me. They say thank you. I don't know what to say beyond that, and the crowd is moving outside to continue marching.

I'm left feeling empty. My poster board sign feels silly and meaningless. Surely there's more I can do.

But this is not about me; the fight is not about my feelings. It's no one's job to make me feel good about what I do in fighting the systematic oppression of minority groups. In fact, that's part of the problem: People in the majority group often want credit for the gestures they make in support of the minority group. I didn't do anything special by approaching those women and giving them hugs. All I did was, for a few seconds, approach them as human beings. This should be the bare minimum of how we interact with each other.

What that interaction at the airport showed me was that I have a lot more work to do on myself before I can be an effective agent of change around the issues facing our country right now. I need to make sure that I'm fully integrated, that I've accepted and acknowledged my white privilege on the deepest level, and that I'm continuously checking my own ego and needs in support of those who deserve a voice. It's long-term process, and a necessary one. But there's simply no other choice.

Because in the end, we're all in this together.

CHAPTER 8

IT'S NOT OKAY

Trigger Warning: Sexual Assault

I said yes. At first.

I was a virgin, and he knew it. He knew I wasn't on birth control, so condoms were a must. I couldn't risk jeopardizing my future—a full scholarship at the University of Alabama and graduate school ambitions—with an unwanted pregnancy.

He entered me, and it hurt. I told him it hurt and asked him to slow down, but he didn't. I laid there and waited for it to hurt less. He said it would get better if we kept going.

He pulled out and took the condom off. He re-entered me. I said no. No, please, stop. I was too drunk and he was too big to push away.

"You need to know what a real penis feels like inside you," he said.

I was 19. He was 33.

As I write this, I'm 33 years old. Nineteen-year olds look like children to me.

He told me that I was "mature for my age," so that made it okay.

He spent the summer buying liquor and getting me drunk. Blackout drunk, night after night. I drank so much I started sleepwalking. I would wake up standing in the hallway or on the second-story balcony. It's like my brain knew the situation was wrong and was trying to help me escape.

He made all the decisions. How much I drank. That I was "mature enough." That I needed to feel a "real penis" inside me. He never asked me what I thought. His opinion was more important than mine.

I told one person. My best friend at the time. I told her I'd lost my virginity, but that the way it happened was wrong and felt bad. She said, "Well, I talked to you that night, and you were pretty drunk. So that's kind of your fault." I didn't tell anyone else for years.

I didn't call it rape for a long time after that.

But I do now. It's taken a very long time and a lot of therapy. But I call it what it is now.

I was raped, and it was wrong. I was manipulated over a series of months into a situation I should not have been in by a person who didn't have my best interest at heart. I was young and naive and inexperienced. I said yes, then no, and that no should have been honored. It wasn't. And that was wrong.

I kept silent for a long time, and the secret ate away at me. It brought a fear to my relationships that I couldn't name or understand. It convinced me that I was unimportant, and that no one would listen if I spoke up, anyway. In all of my writing and blogging about deeply personal aspects of my life, I never mentioned it, because it felt like something to be ashamed of.

But I'm not ashamed now. I recognize the young, vulnerable girl I was and how I was taken advantage of. I don't recognize that as a victim, but as a survivor. It was another storm I weathered, and I'm stronger and more self-aware for it.

I didn't share my story for a long time, although I wanted to. By the spring of 2016, I had done enough work around my rape that I started looking for opportunities to finally share it publicly.

I started to share my story when the Stanford rape case dominated headlines. Many women shared their own stories, and I felt the pull to unburden myself in public, to speak out and be yet another vocal survivor. But I didn't. I wasn't ready yet. I had a few more wisps of a very old shame to brush off and a few more deep breaths to take before I could expose my deepest wound.

But then, in October of 2016, a recording surfaced of the man who would become president in a month, talking about forcing himself on women. A man who was in a position of power and older than the women he pursued, just like the man who manipulated me and forcibly took my virginity. A man who felt his desire was and is more important than the women he's in the room with. A man for whom women mean so little, he believes "you can do anything" to them.

I am those women.

And it's not okay.

His comments are not "locker room banter" or idle chit chat between two men. They are an accurate reporting of behavior and beliefs. This man who could lead us did violate women and does believe he has a right to do so. This man does not respect people. He is not a leader. He is a heartless criminal.

He is a rapist.

And if you choose to deny that fact, you are complicit in the rape of women like me.

Part of my healing process has always been to "do" something with my pain and help others in similar situations. After my recovery from a long-term eating disorder, I became a therapist for people in eating disorder recovery. As a yoga teacher, I talk openly about body image and healing on the mat. I realized earlier this year that it was time for me to do something with the pain of rape that I had felt for so many years.

A few months before the recordings surfaced, I signed on to volunteer with the Rape Response program at the Crisis Center in my hometown of Birmingham, AL. Through that program, I act as an emotional support first responder for people who have been raped. My job is not to fix or counsel, but just to be present, to validate and give information, and, most importantly, to say, "I believe you. And it was wrong." I've only worked a handful of cases so far, but it has already been one of the most rewarding experiences of my life, and I know I will volunteer with Rape Response for a long time. I wish I had had that kind of validation and support when I was raped 15 years ago. I wish all survivors did.

I no longer say my rapist's name out loud, and I won't deign to type the name of the man who believes his status gives him the right to treat women like objects and invalidates the need for consent, regardless of whether or not he is president. But that man has access to the federal funding that keeps programs like Rape Response running. Will he care enough to make sure that money continues to support sexual assault survivors? Can we be certain that all people who experience rape will have a place where they are heard, believed, and validated?

I'm heartened by the resistance movement around the current administration and its ability to block some of the cruel and heartless policies that have already been proposed. This is a fight we have to keep fighting.

We have to show him, once and for all, that "no" means no.

CHAPTER 9

GIVING BACK: TURNING PAIN INTO EMPOWERMENT

Trigger Warning: Sexual Assault

She is 19. She woke up at a party, naked, with bruises on her breasts. She has no idea who drugged her drink. She's not pressing charges.

She's 33. We're the same age, and our birthdays are 4 days apart. She met a man at a gas station who took advantage of her friendliness. All she wants to do is go home and sleep.

She's 15. Her parents found out she was having sex with her 18-year old boyfriend. They couldn't fathom their sweet little girl having sex, so they went to the sheriff. They're pressing charges for statutory rape. She cries in my arms as she tells me he's the only person who's ever cared about her. She knows she'll never see him again.

The first time I worked a case for Rape Response, I was hooked. It's not that I loved hearing rape stories; rape is a horrible, violent crime, and any report of it disturbs a rational and compassionate mind. What hooked me was the opportunity to be present with people who had just experienced rape, to listen to them, validate their experiences, and share with them the hope that healing is possible.

I couldn't have volunteered with Rape Response five years ago. Back then, I didn't even call what happened to me "rape." For the first few years after it happened, I referred to it only as "how I lost my virginity." I bought into the myth that, because I initially consented, I was complicit in what happened. After a few years, I was able to call it "sexual assault." And finally, after years of therapy and trauma work, I was able to call it what it really is: rape.

It was only after I came to accept my own story that I was able to offer back to other survivors. Just minutes after I felt strong in my recovery from the trauma of rape, I applied to volunteer with Rape Response through the local Crisis Center. Volunteering with them means meeting survivors at the center and supporting them as they undergo their rape kit examination and providing information about on-going support services. Mostly, it means hearing and validating their story and helping them begin to process this horrible thing that has happened to them. Rape Response is open 24 hours a day, so sometimes we get calls in the middle of the night to meet a survivor. No matter what time I get a call, I'm always eager to jump in the car and go support someone in need.

I hear bits and pieces of my own story in the stories of the women I support at Rape Response. Many know their attacker, like I did. Many were plied with alcohol or taken advantage of while they were drunk, like I was. Some were taken advantage of by a person in a position of power, like I was. Regardless of the details, we all share the same emotional experiences: shock, fear, shame, self-blame, guilt, anxiety, and sadness. We are united by the impact the violation of rape has in our lives.

The difference in their stories is that, through some great act of Universal grace, they are able to make it to a place that's specifically designed to meet their needs. From the time they arrive at Rape Response, they are told, "I believe you, and what happened to you was wrong." In a society that often dismisses or minimizes the stories of rape survivors, hearing these words can accelerate their healing process by years. They are given medical care, preventative treatment for common STDs, and the morning after pill, all of which help alleviate some of the common practical anxieties women have after sexual assault. And they are given access to free, on-going counseling to address the trauma symptoms of rape. It's impossible to overstate what a difference these factors make at the beginning of someone's healing process.

I've seen women emerge from the bathroom at Rape Response after a shower looking like different people than when they arrived, faces clean, eyes brighter, jaws set with determination as they walk back out into the world. Not a victim, but a survivor.

Being raped will no doubt be the worst experience of a person's life. It's a 10 out of 10 on the "horrible shit" scale. But if a survivor can come to Rape Response and receive a little bit of care, be told that their pain and fear are valid, and know that resources are available--if we can tag a little bit of tenderness and caring onto that horrible memory--perhaps that experience drops from a 10 to a 9.8. And that .2 points creates a small wedge where hope and healing can get in. And the opportunity to offer that to someone is worth getting out of bed in the middle of the night.

Every time I meet a survivor and support them through the first few steps of their healing process, I heal a little inside, too. I didn't have that kind of support and validation in the days after my rape; that didn't come until many years later. But when I offer support to another person--when I meet their eyes and say, "I believe you, and you are not alone"--I re-write pieces of my own story. I, too, transform from a victim to a survivor.

This is a simple truth: The place that has broken in you is the very place from which you can heal others. Because you have compassion for those feeling a similar pain, you can be a powerful healer and helper for those with stories like yours. We must do our own healing work first, so that we greet others from a place of strength. And from that place of strength and understanding, we can have a huge impact on the lives of others.

As a Rape Response advocate, I'm not allowed to tell clients about my personal experience. And I wouldn't, anyway; that time is about them, not me. But my hope is that my deep compassion and understanding for their pain and fear will come across in everything I say and do. I hope that it is an unspoken undercurrent in our interaction and provides some small reassurance that survivors can take with them when they go.

Most survivors will apologize for something at some point in our time together. Whether it's for having us come in on a weekend, or taking up so much time, or simply being there at all. I understand this need to apologize and always try to make sure the client knows that it's okay that we're there together. "There's no need to apologize," I'll say. "I'm happy to be here with you."

CHAPTER 10

FOR THE GIRLS

I hit the back button on my phone. Those first piano chords strike, and my heart melts a little, just like it has every time I've played it today. That first intimate "Hello" that sounds so vulnerable and questioning, yet resigned and self-assured. The way she splashes into the first notes of the chorus like a child cannonballing into the deep end of a pool. Even the way she pronounces the titular word as "Hallo." It all rips me apart in the best way possible.

It's November of 2015, and I've been waiting for Adele's new song for a long time. I loved her last album, 21; it was my solo hiking music for a full year. I love her vulnerability and subtle sassiness. I love how she doesn't fear her dark side and balances it with moments of casual, breezy sensuality. She's confident in sharing her insecurities in a way that feels deeply authentic. And those pipes.

So, yeah. I love her. And I love her new single.

"Hello" arrived during a remarkably girl-power year for women in the media. Feminist icons Sleater-Kinney released a comeback album, and bad-ass-of-the-moment Amy Schumer wrote and starred in one of the biggest movies of the year. Local heroine Britney Howard of Alabama Shakes is pretty much everywhere you look, rocking an extraordinary vocal range and unbeatable stage presence. My personal favorite, Florence + the Machine, released a new album in June that spoke to feeling heartache without letting it disempower you. Facebook was flush with articles about wage gaps and the unfairness of policing women's behavior. I won't go so far as to say it's a great time to be a woman (we'll get there one day!), but it certainly seems as though women's relationship with the media is beginning to shift.

In a cultural climate where women are typically celebrated only as sexual objects--and ignored when they aren't attractive enough to meet that standard--the radical notion that women might be people, too, is beginning to gain some traction.

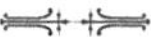

I haven't always had the most comfortable relationship with being female. As a teenager and young adult, I gravitated towards friendships with guys. I loved being the girl who was cool enough to hang out with all the dudes. We went rock-climbing and drank beer in their trucks. They loved my adventurous spirit, and I loved the feeling of approval I felt being the only chick in the crew. A male friend once said in front of a group of other dudes, "Melissa Scott, like, transcends womanhood"; I'm a little ashamed to admit that I took the statement as a compliment.

Looking back, it upsets me that I found joy in rejecting my femininity. I thought being not-girl made me better and more lovable. I found approval through what I was not, rather than what I actually was.

Then college happened, and I found brilliant professors and mentors who introduced me to feminism and social justice. They showed me not only the ways women are oppressed in society but also the ways we internalize that oppression. They gently challenged me to question assumptions I made about being female. I realized that I'd internalized the notion that being male was better, which led me to seek out relationships with men and value them over connections with women. This was self-oppression, and I'd been doing it for a long time.

As I embraced recovery from my decade-long eating disorder, I realized how much of that oppression I'd taken on and recreated in my own internal life. I believed I was not good enough as I was--in part because I thought my value came from being "skinny" and attractive--so I needed to alter and control my body to be "better." And I didn't want to live that way anymore. Most of my intimate relationships were still with men, but I began to entertain the idea that it was time to let women--and the acceptance of femininity--into my life.

In graduate school for Counseling, I folded into a world dominated by women. Not just women, but touchy-feely, lovey, supportive therapist types who took me under their wings and supported me for being the exact person that I am. I began to open up to women for the first time in my life. I was vulnerable and raw about my struggles and insecurities. And I was deeply accepted and loved for it.

And then, on the eve of my 30th birthday, I set off the bomb that would dismantle my life: I told my husband I wanted a divorce. I'd never not had a man by my side, and now I was actively choosing to go it alone for a while. Women from all over reached out to me, letting me know they'd been there and validated both my fear and my strength. My female friends huddled around me, wiped my tears, and propped me up until I could walk on my own again. And when I could, I discovered I still wanted them close.

Now, I savor my relationships with women in my life. I seek out women for both friendship and professional collaboration. Nothing excites me more than power lunching with a fellow bad-ass female and dreaming up an inspiring new project, perhaps after an hour or so of comparing notes on life and love and other important stuff.

When women unite, a force takes over. Women who embrace their power light up in the presence of other women. We become creative and authentic and inspired. It is with women that you can be vulnerable and strong at the same time. My beloved male friends say, "I care about you." My female friends say, "I get you."

And in return, I say, "I need you."

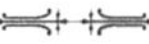

I drool over the track list of forthcoming songs on <u>25</u> as I pre-order on iTunes. The release date can't get here soon enough. As I embrace my own womanhood and find greater joy in welcoming women into my life, female artists seem to write the soundtrack of this new chapter of my life. It seems fitting that my internal journey is outwardly reflected back to me as mainstream feminism gains traction and more women dominate the media on their own terms.

In announcing her new album on her website, Adele is characteristically both self-deprecating and self-accepting. She knows that critics and fans alike have wondered when she'll ever release her next work. She manages to apologize unapologetically, acknowledging others' wait time while validating her own experience.

"I'm sorry it took so long," she says. "But you know, life happens."

Nothing to apologize for, sister. You're right on time.

CHAPTER 11

WE GO HIGH

On November 9th, 2016, I sat--like so many people did--in a state of shock: sad, confused, defeated. Exhausted from almost no sleep. Deeply hurt and betrayed. And very, very scared.

It's hard to deny that the world changed on that election night. And I don't say that in a "boo hoo, I didn't get by way" sense. I mean we elected a man whose statements and values align closer to foreign dictators our country has fought against than the principles of freedom and respect so many have fought for. We had a dream of a country in which the rights of women, people of color, LGBTQIA+ individuals, and people of various faiths would continue to advance. And it seems that in one unexpected swoop, that vision has been swept aside in favor of an America that is fear-based, hate-filled, and overwhelmingly white.

We have no choice but to accept that this is the man who will lead us for the next four years. We don't have to like it or support it, but we must accept it. It is the reality we will live in. And as we grieve, we face inevitable decisions about how to move forward.

So how do we build a nation of hope and love and equality under the leadership of a man who values none of those things?

For me, the answer is simple.

Mr. President, we will do it without you.

You don't want to welcome Muslim people into our country? Fine. We will create spaces where Muslim people feel like welcomed and valued parts of our communities. People of other faiths will attend services at mosques and get to know our Muslim neighbors. We will celebrate them and the beautiful diversity they bring to our country.

You want to deny rights to LGBTQIA+ people? Fine. We will celebrate the members of that community and march through the streets with rainbow flags held high, so that you never forget that they and their allies are citizens of this country, too. We will fight in our own institutions, like our workplaces, to decrease discrimination and increase visibility and social justice. We will raise our children to know that they live their lives however they see fit and love whomever they wish, and we will protect them from the kind of bigotry you espouse.

You want to denigrate the lives of people of color and endorse a system in which people are shot for their skin color? Fine. We will gather around our brothers and sisters of color and speak out against such atrocities every time they happen. We will document with video when we can, and take to the street every time another black or brown person dies so that you never forget that we believe their lives matter.

You want to repeal women's rights, objectify our bodies, and openly treat us with disrespect? Fine. We will stand stronger in our truth and celebrate our feminine strength. We will run for office on the state, local, and national levels until you are so surrounded by strong, forward-thinking women that you have no room to hide behind your cries of "locker room talk" and misogynistic dismissals.

You want to bully people who don't agree with you? Fine. We will be so extraordinarily kind to each other, your angry words will sound like nothing at all. You will fade into the background, looking like a relic from a darker, less-enlightened, more hate-filled era of our history.

One thing is certain: We cannot give in to defeat. We cannot back down from the extraordinary fight that lays before us. We cannot let fear overcome the love we have for one another and the basic belief that all lives deserve dignity, compassion, and respect.

In this time of darkness, sadness, and confusion, we must turn toward each other. We must remember the things that bring us together and recognize the beauty and fire in each others' hearts. We must unite our voices and our actions to create the future we've dreamed of all along.

Remember what she said.

We are stronger together, my friends.

PART THREE:

Life

CHAPTER 1

NOTES FROM THE ROAD

Cooper looks at me from his carrier. His eyes are big and green and calm. He's done and seen this all before. He's got the mix of curious and knowing that seasoned travelers wear.

I'm just delighted to see a cat in the Atlanta airport.

His mom pulls him out, and he sits calmly in her lap. She lets me pet him. This is his 2nd cross-country trip in his 10 months of life. The last was a 12-hour drive from Chicago to Philly. He handled it like a champ and spent a clandestine night in a no-pets-allowed hotel.

He is less bothered by the turbulence than the rest of us.

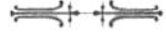

"If there is a doctor on board, we need your assistance at this time," the flight attendant says over the intercom. "We have a medical emergency on board. Again, if there is a medical doctor on board, please ring your flight attendant call button."

A tall man with glasses and a Mets hat rises and motions to the flight attendants. He stands in the aisle talking to a passenger for a little while before eventually sitting down next to him. The flight attendants bring oxygen and a first aid kit. There's a lot of activity for a little while, then it all stops.

"Please remain seated when we reach the gate. Paramedics are meeting us there and will assist a passenger off the plane. Once they have exited, you will be allowed to gather your things and de-plane."

The tall man with glasses and a Mets hat stays on the plane with the flight attendants while the rest of us exit. I never know--I will never know--what happened to the gentleman he sat next to.

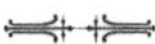

Tasha moved to Phoenix two and a half years ago. A year ago, she left her corporate job to start a cake decorating business, which is going well. She misses her family in the Bronx, but she likes the Arizona sunshine. Like a lot of people, she drives for Uber on the side for a little extra cash.

She was in Manhattan on September 11th, just a few blocks from the World Trade Center. She heard the towers collapse. She and a friend walked two miles up town, where they were picked up by a another friend with a car. It took them over three hours to get home. None of them spoke on the way home that day. There was simply nothing to say, she said.

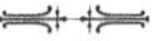

Miss Annie is 83 years old. She's dressed in a turquoise pants suit, brown heels, and a fuchsia manicure. She's flying solo from Phoenix to Atlanta to celebrate her daughter's retirement. She will stay for three weeks. Her main goal on the trip is to celebrate. Her daughter is meeting her at the airport with a gin and tonic in a thermos. Miss Annie has marijuana edibles in her bag.

"I didn't put my teeth in. I came to party!" she says.

Chris has been driving for Uber since August. Last Friday, he picked up a man whose wife had just kicked him and his dog out of the house. The man stood in the rain crying while he waited for Chris to get him. He directed Chris to a bad part of town, where the man picked up a prostitute and went to an hourly motel with her. He paid Chris $50 to wait outside. The dog waited in the car, too. When the man came back to the car, he said, "I just wanted to feel loved for a minute."

Chris's own wife moved out of state last year. They're still married. She took the only paid-for car they owned, leaving him with two car payments and the care of their three children. She doesn't send home any money to help out. Occasionally, she comes back to town to ask Chris for money.

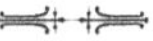

I hear them coming before I see them. A family of ten--five adults and five children--up the stairs of the Mega Bus headed back to Birmingham. They fill the seats on all sides of us with their bodies and their noise. There's a lot of profanity. They pass children back and forth between the seats. One older lady appears have a hard time breathing, but no one in their group seems especially concerned with it. One young woman has everyone's attention. She's visibly drunk and worse and has an ace bandage wrapped around her elbow. She alternates between passing out on her seat mate and stumbling up and down the aisle yelling at people about nothing.

The driver kicks her off the bus before we leave the station.

Everyone quiets not long after we hit the interstate. The bus goes dark, and most people go to sleep.

I look at the children around me. Their tiny bodies are curled in on themselves, reclined on and surrendered to the forms of the only adults they know. I wonder what their lives are like. What are they learning from the big people in their lives? Will they finish school and have careers and love themselves and make good choices? Am I imposing my values on them? Would I worry about them less if they--or the adults in their lives--had skin the same color as mine?

I say a prayer and thank God for putting me face-to-face with my own prejudices. I can only change my biases when I confront them.

I ask for the blessing of travel for as long as I live. Please let me see many faces in my life. Please let me hear many stories.

⚡

It's 1am, and the bus is silent. I questioned the wisdom of taking the bus over staying overnight in Atlanta. Until we crest the hill and see the lights of downtown Birmingham, glistening and fluorescent and familiar. It will feel so good to sleep in my own bed tonight.

I say another prayer of gratitude. Thank you, God, for a home to come back to. Please help me remember the lessons learned on the road.

I check my email one more time as we wait for a final Uber ride, the one that will take me back to the softness of my memory foam mattress and comfort of purring cats next to my head.

An email from AirBnB. "DON'T FORGET! You have a reservation coming up in Austin, TX in two weeks!"

I smile. I haven't forgotten, I think. Let me get a good night of sleep. I'll be ready to head out again soon.

CHAPTER 2

ON GIVING NO FUCKS: LIFE AFTER 30

I've never understood the cultural convention that turning 30 is the end of something, that it's an event to be mourned, the death of youth. Turning 30 is one of the best things to ever happen to me. I believe that wholeheartedly and will tell anyone who will listen.

When I turned 30, I quit giving a fuck. I stopped caring what people think about me. I stopped living my life in a way that looked nice on the outside and started living in a way that felt good on the inside. I took huge career risks without caring what my family or friends thought about my unconventional decisions. I quit following trends and started wearing clothes I like, regardless of what's in fashion. I started telling off men who told me to smile on the street. I started standing up to people who are rude to me and calling out bad behavior. And I got really comfortable running into the grocery store in my pajamas.

My 30s have been amazing so far, but you wouldn't know that from hearing the story of where I was on my 30th birthday. In reality, it was one of the darkest, hardest times in my life.

On March 2nd of 2013, my then-husband moved out of my house. I was alone for the first time in my life, and solely responsible for the home we had bought together. On March 18th, just 16 days later, a freak 15-minute storm blew through Birmingham and knocked over a 45-foot tall oak tree in my backyard, sending it into power lines and ripping all the electrical connections off my house. I came home at sunset to find power company employees in my backyard, casually informing me that I had a "huge problem." I had been on my own for just over two weeks, and I was literally powerless.

On March 20th, I turned 30.

I woke up on the morning of my 30th birthday away from home, unmoored and overwhelmed by the constant flurry of phone calls with insurance companies and contractors. The night the tree fell, I'd spent about 12 minutes in a "someone please take care of me, I need an adult" panic before shifting into "let's get this shit taken care of" mode. I heard myself on the phone negotiating with my insurance agency and taking contractors to task for not showing up on time, skills I didn't even know I had and tasks my ex-husband would have handled in the past. I felt myself digging deep into a new layer of "bad bitch" I'd never needed to access before. Despite the uncertainty and chaos surrounding me, I woke up on my birthday morning focused on doing what I needed to do and getting it done no matter what.

My birthday is the first day of spring, and I've always loved poetic symbolism of rebirth as I celebrate the coming of a new year. Here I was, truly in a new season of life, one that dawned with a new internal fire. I felt lit from within. I was turning 30 with power and gusto. This new decade of life brought intense new challenges, but also some intense new realizations about what I was capable of handling.

Some time before contractors hauled away the great, grand oak tree that had crash-landed in the middle of the new chapter of my life, I went outside and spent some time with it. I sat next to it for a while, staring at it, studying it, in awe of its mass and solidity. And, because I'm a hippy-dippy yoga type who anthropomorphizes objects around me, I asked it a question.

"What are you here to teach me?"

And, because I'm a hippy-dippy yoga type who sometimes gets messages from the anthropomorphized objects around me, I heard it answer.

"I'm here to show you that you're stronger than you think you are. You already know that. You say it. But I'm here to show you that that Truth is so much bigger than you think. You can handle more than you've ever imagined. And you'll be fine. Don't doubt yourself. You're going to be okay, no matter what."

And because I'm a hippy-dippy yoga type who feels the anthropomorphized objects around me are full of wisdom, I believed it.

The intervening years have been far from perfect. Each new spin around the globe has brought an intense new challenge. At least one moment every year, I find myself curled up in bed, crying so hard I'm afraid I might bust a lung, uncertain how or if I'll be able to go on. But every time, I get up, dust myself off, and keep moving forward, secure in the knowledge that I'll ultimately be just fine.

It's not that I don't still struggle sometimes. It's simply that things that used to render me helpless don't seem like that big a deal anymore.

Financial insecurities that used to keep me up at night now just feel like bumps in the road, and I trust that I'll always be able to provide for myself.

Break-ups that would have ripped me apart in my 20s are now simply reset buttons, opportunities to reconnect with the essence of who I am and what I want out of life.

When I hear about people talking negatively about me or my teaching--something that would have shredded my self-esteem in my 20s--I'm now able to shrug it off and remember that I don't live my life to make other people happy.

Perhaps the reality of giving no fucks in my 30s is simply the knowledge and confidence that, no matter what, I'm going to be totally and completely okay.

As write this, I'm just a few weeks out from my 34th birthday. Turning 34 will officially put me in my mid-30s. I like the idea of being in the middle. I'm far from where I started this decade, and I still have a long way to go. My 30s don't look anything like I thought they would. In some ways, they're a whole lot better.

At 34, I own both a home--my second on my own--and a successful small business. I have no debt other than my mortgage, and I travel almost as much as I'd like to. The day after my 34th birthday, I'll get on a plane to Argentina to spend 10 days traveling solo, an idea that would have intimidated me five years ago, but now sounds like exactly how I want to spend the first week and a half of my new year.

As someone who spent her 20s overcoming near-debilitating perfectionism, I simply don't have a lot of fucks left to give to what other people think about me. I've been through a lot, life is weird and tiring, and I'd rather save my energy for things that bring me joy. And as I enter the middle of this decade of internal freedom and strength, I'm excited to see how each new year of life will unfold.

CHAPTER 3

THE BREAK-UP SUITE

My 30s thus far have been punctuated by a series of challenging relationships and devastating break-ups. When I dismantled my life in my divorce at age 30, I knew I was stepping out into a world of new possibilities, new loves, and new people. What I found was a shocking amount of humanity and lessons about the human heart.

The iconic spiritual text <u>A Course in Miracles</u> teaches that every relationship, romantic or otherwise, is a "holy assignment." Whether we pass or fail is determined solely by whether we learn the lesson we are meant to learn from that person. If we choose not to, or if we walk away without internalizing that unique lesson, then we will be confronted with it in our next relationship, and the next, until we finally take in what we are meant to know about ourselves and about love.

This has certainly been the case for me. Each man I welcomed into my world brought unique lessons and experiences. I learned that love is never easy. I learned that it requires both partners to work equally hard. I learned that some people, no matter how much we love them, are only meant to be in our lives for a short time.

But most of all, I learned about myself. Specifically, that I am good enough on my own, and I don't need anyone to complete me.

Some of my favorite pieces I've ever written happened after break-ups. And so here, I've compiled them in honor of the holy assignments of my 30s and the men that came with them.

Thanks, guys. This one's for you.

February 2013: Yoga for a Broken Heart

This is the piece I've been avoiding writing. This is the one I've been agonizing over for weeks. The one that brings me to tears every time I sit down to write it. The one I've been fearful of writing and, mostly, of posting. This is The Big One.

I'm getting divorced.

It didn't happen suddenly. There was no anger and no major blow-ups. No betrayal or hurt. No accusations or yelling. It was a rational decision made by two adults who love each other and want what's best moving forward.

And it sucks.

He's been my best friend for a long time. He's my rock and my safe place. When we first started dating, I was freshly in recovery from my eating disorder, had just moved back to the South after a grueling stint in Chicago, and had absolutely no idea what direction I was headed next. He grounded and supported me as I entered graduate school and went through yoga teacher training. He introduced me to martial arts and showed me that my body could be strong. He taught me how to laugh again and re-connected me to my love of nature. He told me I was beautiful every single day until I believed it, and then kept telling me because he believed it so much. He helped me grow, heal, and come back to life. And he tells me I did the same for him.

Seven years later, we still love each other, but in a different way. We've loved each other through so much growth that we're very different people now than we were back then. We've helped each other grow into the people we're meant to be... and now it's time for us to go off and be those people. We're letting each other go with love and each other's sincerest blessings.

I'm crying a lot. Big, hot tears that well up in the car and in public restrooms when I'm not expecting them at all. It's a hard thing to talk about when people ask me, and even harder to initiate conversations about. I get caught off guard by how sad it is. Some days all I want to do is curl up in bed and cry.

Thank God for my yoga practice. As my whole world comes unhinged, my mat has once again become the ground beneath my feet. I come to my mat now to remind myself that everything is okay. My practice at once familiar and exhilarating as I remember the strength my body holds. The strength I feel in my arm balances and Fists of Fire lunges reminds me that I can get through anything. I can hold and support myself.

And sometimes I come to my mat for release. I feel a lump in my throat or an aching in my chest, and I know there's something there that needs to be moved out. So I move through a few salutations and wait for the tears to come. And when they do, I crumple into Child's Pose and let them flow. I do my best crying ujayi and whisper to myself, "This too shall pass, this too shall pass..."

It's times like this when we're called to truly walk the yogic walk. I have to self-nourish and self-nurture, just like I tell my yoga students to do. I have to show up honestly and allow authentic expression to happen, no matter what it looks like. And I have to trust. Trust myself, trust the Universe, and trust the process. I have to stop and breathe. And breathe. And breathe.

I honestly don't know what's on the other side of all this, just like I never know what's on the other side of the next pose. As I move into my thirties as a single woman and face the daunting task of solo home-ownership, I could fall flat on my face. And I have to be okay with that. If I do, I'll pick myself up and try again, just like

I do in my practice. Or maybe I'll stop and rest and re-group until I'm ready to try something different.

And I'll pause for a moment to offer gratitude. In this hardest of transitions, I'm so grateful for all those who support me, for those who call and text, for those who hold me in lingering hugs when they see me and say, "I've been thinking about you." I'm grateful for my family who send Facebook messages reminding me I always have a place to stay. And for my brother who texts me jokes to cheer me up and let me know he's thinking of me. And for my Dad, who emails to tell me he's always there for me, no matter what.

And for you (you know who you are), I am so, so thankful. Thank you for everything you've ever done. I love you, and I always will. Namaste.

December 2014: A Tale of Two Christmases

On a cold Sunday in December of 2012, I walked into the sanctuary of Dawson Memorial Baptist Church, alone in a crushing sea of well-dressed worshippers and adorable young families. An usher stopped me.

"How many?" he asked.

"Just me," I said. I clutched the handkerchief in my pocket, already fighting back a swell of tears.

"Just you?" he replied. "I have one seat left right up front. Come with me!"

He whisked me through the crowd to the front of the church. There was one seat left on the second row, behind the seats reserved for church elders and other very important types, next to a beautiful family with three children, all blond and startlingly well-behaved. "Lucky you!" the usher said, gesturing to my unexpectedly VIP seating. "Enjoy!"

I sat down next to the young blond father of the young blond family who would be my pew-mates for the next two hours. I felt terribly underdressed, in my jeans and ponytail, amongst church-goers in their Christmas finest. But I let myself off the hook, knowing that it was a Christmas miracle that I was there at all.

I started to lean over to the blond father next to me and whisper, Please forgive me for all the crying I'm going to do. But I stopped myself. There was no one to apologize to for what I was going through.

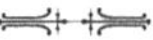

Two days before I entered the church for their annual Christmas Candlelight Service, my husband and I had decided to separate. Our timing was terrible. We had wrapped presents for family members under the tree and dear friends coming to stay with us from out of town the next week. For reasons I don't remember now, it made the most sense at the time to tell no one we were divorcing until after the holidays. So I found myself totally alone, in crushing isolation, facing the scariest transition I'd ever considered, and having to keep it a secret. I knew the coming months would be horrifically dark, and I was clinging to faith that there was light on the other side. My husband and I weren't angry at each other, which almost made the inevitable loss of him even harder. We were still sharing a bed and still had gifts to give each other, knowing it would be the last time we celebrated a holiday together. I sat the pew feeling engulfed by a terrifying limbo.

Even as I fought the urge to run out of the church to sit in my car and cry some more--as I had taken to doing on an almost daily basis recently--I knew I needed to be there. Church had stopped being the place I connected with the Divine many years ago, but in this state of raw vulnerability, I needed something familiar. I needed to be surrounded by the wholesome sights and sounds of the holiday season that used to feel so magical and safe when I was small. I needed to hear the comforting story of a baby born in a manger on a dark night, bringing the promise of hope and brighter days ahead. I needed to feel the warmth of a community, even though it wasn't my community, and to remember that I wasn't truly alone.

I did cry that night. There in a room full of thousands of strangers, I let the music and the message of hope touch the rawest places of my heart. I whisper-sang along with the Hallelujah Chorus, words and notes I remembered from similar performances in my childhood many years ago, their familiarity a thin balm to the places in me that ached. The blond man next to me was kind in his presence, and did not draw attention to my obvious tears. Perhaps I was projecting, but I swear I even felt compassion radiating from him. I soaked through my handkerchief and, for once, did not judge myself for such an open display of emotion.

The service ended, and families stood and began to maneuver their way out of the beautifully decorated church. I stood off to the side waiting for the crowd to subside. I didn't have the energy to fight my way to the front of the church just yet, and nowhere in particular to go. I waited in the candlelight and pondered the deep aloneness the coming months would bring.

After some time, the crowd thinned, and I picked up my heavy wool coat and slid one arm into a sleeve. The coat slipped away from me, and I struggled to pick up the other side. Suddenly, the weight of it became lighter. I turned to see an older man behind me, holding the other side of my coat in a gesture of gentlemanly compassion. Our eyes met. He smiled.

"Thank you," I said, a bit breathless and stunned. My voice sounded rusty, as if I hadn't spoken to another human being in a long time.

"Merry Christmas," he said. His hand lingered on my shoulder for a moment. A fleeting look of concern crossed his expression as he no doubt took in the tear stains and red blotches on my face.

But then he smiled brighter, his blue eyes shining kindly in the candlelight, as if to say, Whatever it is, you're going to be okay.

The moment lasted no longer than a breath, but in that brief encounter something cracked in me. I was able to hear the message loud and clear: I wasn't truly alone, and there are always those who will pick up and help carry my burdens.

In the months that followed, no truth was more clear to me than that. Once I finally shared the reality of my situation, the gaping void left where my husband used to be was filled by friends and family who checked on me daily, brought me food and small gifts, and reminded me that they were there for me. They listened to me when I needed to talk and told me jokes when I needed to laugh. In one act of superhuman friendship, on a particularly dark Saturday night when I wasn't sure if I could make it to the next morning, my dearest friend Connie actually procured for me the keys to a church so that I could cry gut-wrenching tears in the sanctuary, comforted once again by the familiarity of a house of the Divine. She sat with me until my tears dried and I was able to walk back into the world feeling strong once again.

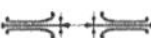

Yesterday, on Christmas Eve, I went to the grocery store to buy last minute ingredients for Christmas Day cooking. My family has had a strange year (a post for another day), so I'm hosting my father and brother for the first time. The strangeness of the year and change in usual holiday schedules meant that I was by myself on Christmas Eve for the first time in my life. I thought I'd be sad about it, but I walked into Publix feeling very happy and excited about both an Eve on my own and a Day with two of my favorite people in my home.

One of my favorite Publix employees stopped me to say hello. He's a older man with kind blue eyes. He always asks me about my day. He's so sweet and genuinely interested in my life, I'm not even bothered that he calls me "sweetie" and "darlin'". I've wondered if he knows about my divorce. He used to greet my husband and me when we shopped for groceries together. I'm sure he's noticed that I shop alone now.

"How ya doin', sweetie? Got any plans tonight?"

"I'm good!" I said. "No plans tonight. Just going to enjoy a quiet evening to myself."

"Just you?" he asked, surprised, a look of concern crossing his face.

"Just me," I said.

"Well, that's no good! No one should be alone on Christmas Eve."

I smiled. "No, it's okay," I said, feeling a swell of gratitude for the truth of what I was about to say. "I might be by myself, but I'm never alone."

April 2014: On Being Public

Recently, within a week of each other, two different people said to me, "You're kind of a celebrity." The first time, I nearly spit out a mouthful of water. The second time, I nearly choked on my panini.

"Well," I said both times, "The nature of my work is very public. And I'm fortunate enough to get to work with some great people." A smooth answer, but on the inside, I was surprisingly embarrassed. A celebrity? Me? Not possible. Celebrities are glamorous and interesting. I'm just a normal chick. I change into my pajamas as soon as I get home every day. I read about nerdy things on the internet. I have a hard time keeping plants alive. I struggle with social anxiety on occasion. I never, ever wear make-up. I'm just a normal, average, slightly boring girl.

My drink and dinner companions were insistent, though. "No, really. People, like, know you. Everyone I know either does yoga with you or knows someone who does. People gush about you."

By this point in the conversation, my Ego had twisted about as far to the left as it could manage and was begging for mercy. I deftly changed the subject. I deflected attention away from myself and onto the other people. Just like I always do.

You see, for all the public-ness of what I do, I've never really been comfortable being the center of attention. I realize that sounds silly coming from someone who stands and talks in front of people for a living, but it's true. People who know me well will stop a conversation and say, "Quit doing that thing where you don't talk about yourself and ask a bunch of questions instead." Some of this is a service mindset. I strive to live my life in service of others and their highest self. But some of it is straight-up fear of being seen, which translates to a fear of being vulnerable.

My very public work actually puts me in the position of being able to hide from truly being seen. I can put the focus on the teaching, the yoga, the student, and--even though I'm the one talking--never actually have any attention on myself. In times of great stress, I often retreat to my work, because it is the safest place to hide without totally isolating myself. Hiding in plain sight, so to speak.

And yet there are times when I can't even hide in my work. Times when my work confronts me with the very thing I'm trying to run from. Last weekend, during a deeply stimulating and emotional conversation with my wonderful teacher trainees, themes of grief and relationships ending kept coming up. I found myself at a complete loss for words. The conversation touched on something too deep, too raw, too fresh within myself to run from in that moment. So, against my better judgment and all my training as a professional, I turned the attention to myself.

"I'm sorry," I said. "I'm struggling with what to say because I'm relating too much. I got dumped last night."

I did not want to say those words. I DID NOT want to admit that I was terribly vulnerable and hurting underneath my confident teacher exterior. It's not that I was faking it, it just felt safer, as it usually does, to focus on the other person, on my beloved students who are looking to me for knowledge and guidance. It usually feels better to focus on them. But in that moment, I needed to turn the focus back on myself. I needed it to be about me. I held my breath waiting for their response, worried that I might lose status in their eyes for bringing my personal stuff into the training room.

But they were amazing. They whispered expressions of sympathy. Some got teary-eyed. When we took a break, they gave me hugs, asked how I was really doing. They brought me little gifts the next day, and sent me texts, emails, and messages as the week wore on. Just checking in, just expressing love.

The most amazing part is that it felt good. Good to be seen and validated in my sadness. Good to feel cared for. Good to be able to be my deeply flawed, deeply human self for a minute. Whatever I had been hiding from wasn't there after all. All that was there--and this shouldn't have surprised me--was love.

Will I quit hiding in my work from now on? Probably not. Old habits don't die that easily. But will I remember to let my guard down and let the people I love return that love to me once in awhile?

Definitely.

October 2014: Anatomy of a Practice

2:58pm

My mat hits the ground with a familiar thu-thunk. The room is still warm from the last class. Every step of getting to this moment is choreographed. The thump of the lock as I enter. The way I take my shoes off and arrange my purse, taking my water bottle out of my bag. I enter the studio quietly, pausing to soak in the silence. Always the same.

This time is sacred. I've been practicing at exactly this time in exactly this spot every week for years. The hour before I have to open the studio for my 4:30 class. The space is usually quiet. It's the middle of my day, and I'm transitioning from one role to the next. The beginning is always the same. Routine creates ritual.

3:03pm

Warm-up. I didn't feel like practicing today. I'm tired. Not just sleepy, but bone-tired, heart-tired. I snake my spine back and forth, feeling my a slight tension in my spinal ligament, a grip between my shoulder blades. Another heartbreak last night, the end of another dream. The beginning was so lovely. I thought maybe I'd found The One…

Despite my mental resistance, my body is asking to move. I'm wearing sadness in my physical form like a cloak, and despite my Ego's desire to cling to it, my wiser self is begging for release. I feel my fascia start to liquify, and I'm able to deepen into the movements. Navasana pulses, Cat-Cow, Down Dog. Shapes so familiar, they're like family members. I settle into the rhythm. Familiarity calms my mind.

3:08pm

Sun Salutations. Breathe in, breathe out. Repeat. Tears creep up and recede. Up Dog, heart opens, chin quivers. Down Dog, shoulders draw protectively around the heart. Damn, I'm sad. I wonder if I should check my phone, maybe he's texted. Maybe I should text him… No. Breathe in, breathe out. Repeat. Stay present, notice your hands and feet on the mat. Ground.

3:16pm

Standing Pose Flow. Lunge, Pyramid, Warrior 2, Triangle. Familiar, rhythmical, soothing. An expression of where I am today, an opportunity to give myself what I need. I feel strength returning to my legs. Standing a little taller now. It takes longer to warm up now than it did ten years ago, but that's to be expected. When I do arrive, the stretch is deeper. I'm able to feel individual threads in my hamstrings that open or resist. Awareness cultivated over years and hundreds of hours of practice. Breathe in, breathe out.

In Half Moon, I crack again. I crumble to the floor for a moment, tears overtake my face, and I'm blinded. Shit, maybe it was the wrong decision. Maybe I should have tried to make it work… No, the timing wasn't right. God, I'm sad… Down Dog. Re-ground. Hands and feet on the mat. Breathe in, breathe out. Start over.

3:21pm

Standing Splits. What's that I always say in class? Keep the foundation strong. Trust your legs to support you. Out of that strength, surrender. Upper body soft. The balance between effort and ease. Dive. Know you are supported.

3:26pm

Bird of Paradise. Hamstrings have finally given way to the extraordinary openness they're capable of. Leg in the air, foot above the head. Standing leg strong. Press down, lift up. I realize that somewhere along the way, I've shed a layer. Breathe in, breathe out.

3:33pm

Handstand. My daily exercise in patience. Has it been three years, maybe, that I've practiced handstand almost every day? Finally able to hold for a breath, maybe two. On occasion four or five. My wide open shoulder joints inevitably betray me, flipping me into a backbend. I watch the frustration rise and fall. It's okay. Lay on the floor for a minute. Recover. Stand back up and try again.

My heart is tired. I've been at this game for so long. Putting myself out there, diving in, trusting. I knew there would be no guarantees when I walked away from something safe and secure. This last one felt so right. Timing. Timing is everything.

Hands down, kick up. Repeat. Trust. Know that you will fall at some point. Lay down for a minute. Recover. Then try again. Don't forget to breathe.

3:39pm

Arm Balances. The practice is finally starting to take. I feel open and strong. Bending into Flying Splits and Eight-Angle Pose. I briefly consider posting a yoga selfie to Instagram. Nah. Today is too private. Today the practice is for me. Breathe in…. Breathe out…

3:41pm

Forearm Balance. My favorite. A pose that eluded me for so long, but now fits my body like a glove. A testament to practice. I glide effortlessly up, as I've done so many times before. One breath I'm on the ground, and the next I'm flying. Suspended between heaven and earth.

I look back at my upside-down reflection in the mirror. I'm sweaty and pink. My belly swells to its full Buddha-ness on the inhale, contracts on the exhale to show abs that will never form a six-pack but are strong nonetheless. Breathe in… breathe out… I feel like I could hang here all day, supported by my own strong shoulders, between which hangs my heart. Perhaps not as tired as I thought it was.

Rest in Child's Pose. Forehead down, third eye supported by the earth. I'm stronger than I think I am. Sweat drips onto the mat. I'm consumed–spontaneously–by gratitude for those who got me to this place, for those who teach me increasingly deeper lessons about my ability to love. I say his name, and thank the Universe for setting him in my path.

3:44pm

Backbend. Full wheel. Heart open. No tears. Watching the sadness rise and fall with my breath. Breathe in… breathe out… It's all okay…

3:52pm

Forward Folds. Melting into easy simplicity. My muscles have unknotted, and my body feels less encumbered, more like mine. I have dissolved into an easier state of being.

A profound sweetness overtakes me. The veil of sadness has lifted, and I am able to look back at the happy moments. The first date where we looked at each other with pleasant surprise, as if to say, where did you come from? The second date on the water, where we walked up to the edge of falling in love and wondered if it was too early. The way we laid in each other's arms and made ourselves laugh almost till dawn. Waking up to love notes and coming home to flowers. Talks about a future that seemed beautiful and bright and full of wonder.

To my surprise, I find the corners of my mouth turned up. My face softens with memory.

Breathe in. Breathe out. My heart is tender, but no longer tired.

3:58pm

Savasana. Tears come again, but this time there's no resistance. They roll off my face and hit my mat with with a delicate tick, tick. I've been here many times before. Not just this pose, but also this place of intense vulnerability. Raw and resting on my mat once again. Somewhere along the way, the sadness transformed from frantic and confusing to something I could wrap my mind and heart around. This too shall pass. This too shall be learned from. This too shall inspire growth.

Rest.

4:01pm

Come up to sit. Groggy, damp with tears and sweat. Relieved. Arms reach up, hands come together at the heart. Ritual, routine. Namaste.

I say the prayer I've said a million times. Thank you, God, for this opportunity to relax and be thankful in my body. I pray for strength and energy and inspiration to teach the best class I can and to give my students what they need.

Today, I pause a moment and add a line to the familiar prayer. I pray for release for myself… and for him. I say his name once again and thank God for the opportunity to learn how to let more love in. I am thankful for him.

4:12pm

The doors are unlocked. I've long since blown my nose and prepared the room for class. Setting the stage for what I have to offer today. The first student arrives, all smiles. "How are you?" she asks.

I pause. I smile a little.

Breathe in.

Breathe out.

"I'm okay," I say.

And I am.

October 2016: Do It Anyway

I don't want to be here. I don't want to give this presentation. I'm exhausted. I only slept two hours last night, up all night replaying the conversation over and over again, whispering out loud the things I'd wish I had said at the time. I have nothing to give right now. I don't want to stand for three hours and talk about small business development. Yes, it's something I'm passionate about. Yes, I know I'll enjoy it once I get started. Yes, I want to do this work and help these people.

But this was our thing. We did it together. Standing here just reminds me of him and he's not here anymore and it's only been twelve hours since he stood in my doorway and told me he loved me for the last time and I don't want to be here and I just want to go back to bed.

I don't want to stand here and be strong and talk about things.

But I'll do it anyway.

I don't want to teach this workshop either. Arm balances and inversions. It's usually my favorite one I do all year. It's light and playful and fun. I don't feel any of those things right now. I feel more flattened than flight-prone. I'm so tired and heavy and confused and it's been less than 24 hours since I told him I wasn't sure if we could even be friends and my heart feels like one big, pulsating bruise.

But these people are here and expectant. They paid for me to show them how to fly. They want me to teach them how to be strong, even though I don't feel strong. They're here with their mats and their intentions, and it's my job to show them how exhilarating getting upside down can be.

I don't feel like I have it in me to lead people toward flight.

But I'll do it anyway.

I don't want to cry all these tears. I don't want to lay in bed and soak tissue after tissue and sob till my stomach hurts. I don't want to feel all the things I have to feel to let him go. I will cry buckets to get him out of my system.

It was all so beautiful once. The things we talked about, plans to travel the world together, projects we wanted to pursue. The way we looked at each other, all soft and starry-eyed. The way we danced and laughed and held each other. The way we always held hands when we walked. The way we traveled well together. The way we called each other "partner." The way other people saw how much we loved each other. The way we knew how much we loved each other.

But it wasn't quite enough. Something never quite fit. He wasn't ready, or maybe I was too ready. Something about it was never the right thing.

I don't want to cry all the tears I need to to let him go.

But I'll do it anyway.

I don't want to think about what comes next. I don't want to move back out into the world single and alone all over again.

Things are different now. Life is different now, and I feel like I'm still figuring out how to navigate this new terrain.

I don't want to put my heart out there yet again, only to attach to a dream of a life, only to perhaps lose that dream all over again.

I don't want to move back out into the world again--when the time is right--to look for love, with my heart wide open and vulnerable and hopeful.

But I'll do it anyway.

I'll do it anyway, because it's the right thing to do.

Because forward is the only direction I know.

I will get up and go out and do what needs to be done.

Perhaps it will hurt. Perhaps I will weep while I walk. Perhaps my steps will look more like stumbles, or for a time, a crawl.

Do it anyway. Do it anyway. Do it anyway. Although you feel defeated, get up and do it anyway. Despite how hard it might feel, do it anyway. Move forward through the hurt and fear and sadness. Make good choices, even when they're hard. Get up when all you want is to lay down. Do it because you can. And you will. And you must.

I don't want to do any of the things I know I need to do to keep moving forward.

But I'll do it anyway.

Because I know that I can.

February 2017: Dear Addiction

Dear Addiction,

I hate you so much.

You are darkness. You eat everything you touch alive, with no remorse. You take everything and twist it into a grotesque version of what it used to be.

You stole a good man from me. A man I wanted to marry, and who--somewhere deep inside--I believe wanted to marry me. You made him ugly and deceitful. You made him petty and unkind and confused. You filled him with shame so thick and black, he couldn't even see me through it. You kept him from feeling my love. You convinced him that he needed bad behaviors to fill the hole you created inside him. You kept him from ever fully sharing his heart with me. You asked him for more and more and more.

You're never satisfied.

As much as I love him, I had to reject you. You created all the secrets and lies that stood between us. You filled me with a fear of him that made me act crazy and say things I didn't mean. You destroyed what we had.

We were going to travel the world together. Our dream was to vagabond, jumping from place to place, seeing everything there is to see, holding hands all the while. We were going to get married in every country in the world. We made each other laugh and danced together and day dreamed. Our love was sweet and playful, tender and joyful.

We loved each other deeply.

Until you destroyed it all.

I had found my partner, the one was I looking for all along. He is kind and sweet and intelligent and funny and loving and thoughtful and generous and spiritual and creative. I see all that is good and bright and right in him. But you hate anything that is good, and you'll stop at nothing to destroy it.

I hope one day you release your grip on him. He deserves so much better than you.

I deserve so much better than you.

Fuck you,
Melissa

Dear Recovery,

I'm so grateful for you.

You are the light in the darkness. You are the path out of addiction. You are hope and faith and healing.

I couldn't save him, though God knows I tried. I was the one who first said the word "addiction." I looked up Twelve Step meetings and told him when to go. I went with him to groups, read books with him, went to counseling with him. I called him out in his narcissistic moments, in hopes of re-finding the beautiful soul inside. I gave him grace when he was defensive. I loved him and held him when he was vulnerable.

And even though he made so many choices that destroyed my trust, my faith, and my self-esteem, thanks to you, I forgave him.

I didn't handle everything well. Some things I did badly. I gave into my fear of his lies and said things I regret. I yelled at him. I asked things of him I shouldn't have in attempt to assuage my pain. I always had the best intentions, but I didn't always act well.

And even though I'm embarrassed by my weak and needful moments and wish I could go back and do it all again, thanks to you, I forgave myself.

Thanks to you, I know that his addiction wasn't my fault. I didn't create it, and I couldn't fix it.

Thanks to you, I know I wasn't crazy, but I was in a crazy-making situation.

Thanks to you, I'm able to still love him from afar.

Thanks to you, I've reclaimed my sense of worth and know that I'm loved and lovable.

Thanks to you, I'm surrounded by a community of women who've been through the same thing and support me unconditionally.

Thanks to you, I have hope that I'll find love again one day.

Thank you,
Melissa

Dear Addiction,
I'm grateful for you.
I never would have chosen you.
But without you, I never would have found Recovery.
And so, I am grateful.

Love,
Melissa

CHAPTER 4

LETTER TO AN OLD HOUSE

Dear sweet House,

Tomorrow your listing will go live. Someone will hit a button and broadcast on my behalf that it's time for me to move on. People will scroll pictures of you. They'll come wander through your rooms. They'll evaluate you, trying to decide if you could feel like home to them. It's an odd thing to think about, strangers in my home. But it's time. You and I both know it's the right thing.

I remember the first night you were mine. Friends helped us move in boxes and furniture. We fed them pizza and gave them jobs to do. And then they left, and for a little while I was here alone with you. I wandered from room to room and sobbed, wondering what on earth I'd gotten myself into. You felt big and empty and hard to fathom. I wondered how I could possibly be responsible for an entire building and the land it sits on.

That was the first time you chuckled at me. I heard you, bemused. "Oh, dear," you seemed to say, "everything is going to be just fine." And for some reason, I believed you. That was the first time you comforted me, but far from the last.

For a little while, you were ours. And later, you became mine. You were the first thing I ever owned completely and fully by myself. There was paperwork to prove it. You were mine, and owning you by myself made me more proud than anything else I'd done to that point. You were little more than empty rooms, but you were my empty rooms, and I knew I would grow into your spaces over time.

Each room I filled in turn filled a little empty piece of my heart. I found pieces of myself in the vibrant colors I painted on the walls. In the turquoise of my bedroom, I found a place to rest. In the green of my yoga room, I found growth and new life. And my favorite, my purple kitchen, represented the abundant life I've been able to create for myself. I filled your walls with art I love and invited friends over to fill the rest with love and good energy. We laughed a lot at those gatherings. Your walls have a way of echoing with laughter for days after friends have left.

You have made me very, very happy. You gave me a place to wait out the darkest days of my life, and a place to celebrate my arrival in some of the brightest. You taught me how to feel strong again, and gave me a place to rest when I was weak.

And now, it's time to move on.

It's time for me to find a space that's just mine from the beginning. I need less to take care of and fewer rooms to clean. Life is pulling me in the direction of increasingly more travel, and I can't give you the care and attention you need. You deserve more than I can give you right now.

But some person or family will be able to give you that. I hope they love you as much as I do.

I will miss you tremendously. I'll miss how quiet you are during the day and how brightly the sunlight shines in your windows. I'll miss the wildness of your backyard that was always the best place to lay and watch the moon. I'll miss the echo of my footsteps on your well-worn wooden floors. I wonder how many times I'll drive in your direction when I'm headed home at the end of the night, before I realize that I'm creating a home in a new place now?

Just like you comforted me that first night, I want to comfort you now. You will be fine. You are big and sturdy and accepting. You have seen many things and will continue to quietly witness the lives that come and go within you and around you. You don't need me to tell you that you'll be okay. You already know that.

Perhaps it's I who need that reassurance from you once again.

At some point, after offers have been made and accepted, and dates have been set, and plans have been made, I'll slip downstairs to the basement. I'll pull out the paintbrush and small container of paint I have set aside. I'll dip the brush and, with tears in my eyes, write my initials somewhere on the unfinished brick of your walls. Small and unobtrusive, in a corner somewhere, I'll leave my mark on you. "Melissa was here." I'll officially become a permanent part of your history.

And as I move on to whatever chapter is next, you'll forever and lovingly be a part of mine.

Love,
Melissa

CHAPTER 5

"YOU'LL NEVER WORK A DAY IN YOUR LIFE"

*"We should catch up! Do you want to meet for coffee at
3:00 on Wednesday?"*
"I can't. That's when I practice."

*"We're going hiking on Saturday afternoon.
Wanna come?"*
"I'd love to, but that's a teacher training weekend."

"How was your day?"
*"So emotional! We talked about what beliefs hold you
back in reaching your potential. Everyone cried. I had to
work so hard to keep the day on track. It was so incredibly
intense... It was awesome."*

We've all heard it: "Do what you love, and you'll never work
a day in your life."
Anyone who's ever chased a dream knows that's total crap.

When I walked away from a well-paying-but-soul-crushing job two years ago to pursue my dream of teaching yoga full-time, I knew I was gambling. I was recently divorced, had a mortgage, and still had a mountain of student loan debt from grad school. My job allowed me to comfortably support myself as a single woman. But it was killing me.

So I jumped. I stepped away from comfort to chase my dream of teaching yoga full-time and leading teacher trainings. And I'm so grateful I did. I love what I do. I get to interact with amazing, heartfelt people every day. I get to design workshops and curriculums that combine the best of what I love. For the most part, I set my own schedule, and most days I stay in my pajamas until 2pm.

My dream-chasing job is amazing, and I love it.

And I've never worked harder in my life.

I wake up in the morning with a mile-long to-do list. I hit the ground running, answering emails, updating teacher training curriculum, putting out new content. Most of the work I do, I don't get paid for directly. Rather, it is an investment in a bigger dream that has provided me with financial abundance for two years. My income comes from events, like workshops that take 2 hours to teach and ten hours to prep. Or teacher trainings that require six months of prep work for a scant 200 hours in-person with my incredible trainees. Every new project is a gamble. Will I put in all this time--time I could work on other things--only to see it fall flat? Or will all my hard work pay off abundantly again?

Moreover, every new project is a deeply personal statement about who I am. "See this? This training is an amalgamation of everything I believe to be important about teaching yoga. It is vulnerable and personal, and I hope you like it." Everything I undertake has as much emotional risk as financial. Everyday is an exercise in courting rejection.

Time and scheduling are constant challenges. Most of my classes, workshops, and trainings happen on evenings and weekends, when my loved ones are free to hang out. I constantly have to say no to invitations because of work obligations.

And I never stop working. At the grocery store, I chat with people about my classes. At parties, I talk to long-time yogis about joining my teacher training. I live my work all day, every day. I never get a chance to turn off.

And in my line of work, the "blood, sweat, and tears" thing is literal. At least the last two are. I hit my mat every day to maintain a steady practice. I flip and fall out of handstand. Sweat drips in my eyes as I flow from Down Dog to plank. I fall out of arm balances and narrowly avoid a faceplant. I practice this way because it makes me a better teacher. I want to understand my students' experience on the mat and teach with compassion. I want my students to know that I'm with them on the journey.

And there are tears. In my teacher trainings, people's "stuff" comes up. I think, in order to be a good teacher, you must recognize the barriers that prevent you from being fully yourself. To stand in front of people and offer something you love is a deeply vulnerable thing. Yoga teachers must do their own personal work to be able to hold space for others. And as the facilitator of that work, I must do my own personal work, as well, doubly so. My career keeps me in constant relationship with my own baggage, in an effort to effectively lead people through their emotional processes.

On top of all that, I always strive for more. There's always another project, another idea, another dream to chase. In 2016, I announced a 300-hour advanced teacher training that I'll lead on top of my yearly 200-hour training. The growth of Birmingham's yoga community excites me, and I hope to see the quality of teaching in the Magic City continue to elevate. I'll do my part to help make that happen.

This is the reality of the dream-chaser. We never turn off. We never finish. We never sit back and rest on our successes. We sacrifice time with loved ones in service of our passion. We take emotional and financial risks to offer what we believe in. We do it because we believe it's worth it.

This yoga teaching gig is the best one I've ever had. It lets me live my dreams. I plan on working hard for what I love for a long time to come. Every single day.

CHAPTER 6

ON FEELING LESS THAN

I read a lot last year. I especially loved <u>Bad Feminist</u> by Roxanne Gay. It's a fantastic book. Gay expertly critiques pop culture, academia, and herself with wry wit and tender vulnerability through a feminist lens that she recognizes as imperfect. About halfway through, my partner at the time asked me how it was, and I responded, "It's the book I wish I had written." Then he gave me a Kindle for my birthday, and the first book I downloaded was <u>Yoga and Body Image</u>, an extraordinary collection of essays by prominent yogis and yoga teachers on how yoga shapes and heals our relationships with our bodies. No, this one, I thought as I read it, THIS is the book I wish I had written.

Mostly, I was just wishing I'd written a book.

Prior to writing this book, I struggled with feeling like I should have written a book already. And why not? I'm an opinionated person with tons of ideas, and "writer" is one of the defining labels of my persona. The comparison demon in my head likes to remind me that people 10 years younger than me have written New York Times bestsellers. Yoga teachers I admire churn out books on topics just outside the periphery of my awareness, as if, given enough time, I could have come up with the same idea, I just didn't get there soon enough. I love to write and I want to write and I plan to write more. Yet here I am, barely pecking out two blog posts a month, nowhere near having written my opus. In this area, I feel like I can't keep up.

Like most women I know, I struggle with feeling less than. Women are conditioned to compare themselves to other women, whether that comparison is fair or not. For example, I'm expected to compare myself to tan, blond, 6 foot tall Giselle Bundchen and buy the products she endorses in an effort to look more like her. At 5 foot 6 with millennia of pasty Irish ancestry at my back and a body that looks soft even at its most fit, a Giselle I will never be. But damned if there aren't an army of marketing execs pushing me to think I should try anyway. A lot of people make a lot of money making women feel "less than."

As options for women have expanded--thrillingly--our less thans have become more complex. In the 80s, my generation's mothers were sold the idea that they could "have it all"-- "all," of course, being a career and a family and a great body and perfect, bouncy hair. In passing this notion down to us, the message morphed from can have it all to should have it all. We should work our asses off to have it all and--thanks, Instagram--make sure we look great doing it and broadcast our multi-layered success for all the world to see.

In this middle of all this I-should-have-written-a-book reverie, I spent some time with a female friend of my then-partner who was in town from Atlanta. To me, she's the epitome of cool. She's a full-time filmmaker with an impressive filmography and constant presence on the film festival circuit. She's currently writing, directing, and producing a 1980s punk rock vintage flick with a mostly female cast. She was in town to screen her latest award-winning, critically acclaimed documentary. She has a cute boyfriend, adorable cats, and an awesome and loving family. She can pull off a plaid shirt better than I ever will. She's always been immensely nice to me, but I've had a hard time getting over the hump of cool-girl intimidation to genuinely connect with her.

"You're, like, my hero," she said suddenly.

I… what?

"I just have so much respect for people who focus their lives on health and wellness. You live a healthy lifestyle and share it with other people and help them. I just think that's amazing. I wish I could be more like that."

I was floored. Here I was, feeling like the nerdy girl at the cool-kid table and this gorgeous, successful woman with the coolest job anyone could imagine was saying she wanted to be more like me. It was an eye-opening moment. She was comparing herself to things I take for granted about my life and--perhaps, although I don't want to make assumptions about her experience--feeling less than. Here we were, two women successful in our fields, admiring each other from across the table and feeling like we had to be less in each other's presence.

Here, of course, is the inevitable question: Why? Why must we do this to ourselves and each other? Why must her inherent coolness morph into a reflection of my perceived--perhaps fabricated--insufficiency?

In writing this, I've just re-read my description of my boyfriend's friend, this inspiring woman for whom I have so much admiration. And something struck me. Is it possible that my description of her isn't so different from how someone might describe me?

She's a yoga teacher with two teacher trainings and a significant presence in the Southeast. She's leading her fourth sold-out teacher training and already getting inquiries about next year's program. She has a cute boyfriend (check), adorable cats (check), and an awesome and loving family (check, and friends). She can pull off yoga pants pretty well, because she has a really nice butt.

Not so bad, right?

There's an old axiom in counseling circles that it's unfair to compare your insides to someone else's outsides. You are privy to your own internal workings, all the negative thoughts, insecurities, and dark moments. No one has access to anyone else's inner experience, so it's easy to assume we're the only weirdos feeling this way. Add to that the glossed-over images on social media, and we're left with the notion that everyone's lives are totally perfect and happy and filled with nothing but delicious brunches and cute puppies.

The title of Roxanne Gay's <u>Bad Feminist</u> comes from two essays in which she bemoans her imperfect dedication to the cause because of things like her love of the color pink and gendered associations with certain household chores. (I don't like killing bugs or taking out the trash, either, sister.) After a number of meditations on how it's pretty much impossible to be a good woman of any kind, given the societal restraints placed on women, she ends her volume with the thought, "I'd rather be a bad feminist than no feminist at all." She'd rather be in the fight, to at least try, than to forfeit and not strive to create a better world of herself and all women.

Gay rejects the notion of being a perfect feminist, embracing the label of "bad," which is really just shorthand for imperfect and human. I'd rather be a bad writer--eking out a few minutes a month to sketch out some mediocre but heartfelt blog posts--than no writer at all. And perhaps Gay beat me to one witty and moving book about feminism, but I trust that there's another one out there, waiting for me to write it. And I trust that when this one comes out, my insecurities will be waiting for me on the other side of that release party. "Sure, you wrote a book, but it wasn't the best book. And you aren't as successful as Liz Gilbert. And that girl on Instagram still has a better handstand than you. And..."

And so on. And as I wrestle my insecurity demons, perhaps other women around me will look to my success as an opportunity to feel less than. I hope they won't, but I know enough about how people work to know someone somewhere probably will. Whoever she is, I hope she realizes that--while she envies me, or a social media star, or whoever else makes her feel less than this week--someone somewhere is admiring how her ass looks in those jeans, or how cute her kids are, or how she manages time for all that volunteer work she does. We're all looking at each other wishing so hard we had the each other's gifts that we forget to be grateful for our own.

My Kindle and I have gotten pretty tight, and I just downloaded Kathryn Budig's new book, <u>Aim True</u>. Kathryn is an amazing international yoga teacher and one of my body image and yoga girl-crushes, so I'm already prepared to wish I had written her book, too. But it's okay. The more I peck out my infrequent blog posts, the closer I get to a book of my own. And when the time comes, I'll be sure to send Roxanne Gay, Kathryn Budig, and all the other women I've compared myself to over the years a free copy, with a note that says, "Thanks being an inspiration, sister."

CHAPTER 7

HOW TO LISTEN

"Will you tell me about her?"

Her eyes widen and fill with tears a little. "Of course!" she says. She seems genuinely surprised I asked. "I'd love to tell you about my sister."

She gestures at the elaborate altar, pointing at pictures and trinkets. She tells me about her younger sister, diagnosed with metastatic breast cancer at age 34. She was given six months to live; she lived another seven and a half years. She tells me about her laughter and spirit. About how she'd never painted before her diagnosis and took up acrylics to process her emotions. Her first paintings were angry and dark; her later paintings become lighter and more reflective. A gorgeous painting of a woman's face sits on the altar. She presented it to my new friend six months before she died.

"This is my first time at Dia de los Muertos, my first time to make an altar for her. She's been gone several years, and I'm ready to tell her story. It's my mission to tell her story now."

I thank her. We hug several times. She tells me I'm part of her Tribe now. I tell her about my own health struggles lately--far less dire than her sister's, but still challenging--and how her sister's story reminds me to be grateful for every day I have.

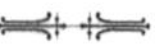

I've always been a Listener. When I was young, I was the friend people came to for advice and support. I held everyone's secrets. For some reason, people found me trustworthy. As I got older, strangers began to open up to me as I made my way through the world. I've held hands in bathrooms with crying women whose names I never learned. I've listened to Waffle House waitresses' custody sagas. I've learned more about strangers' relationship drama in a short elevator ride than their therapists ever did.

I don't mind taking on this role. The truth is, I love to listen. I feel honored when people trust me with pieces of their lives. It's no surprise I sought out graduate training in Counseling; my diploma might as well read "Master of Arts in Listening to People." People who know me well laugh at how easily I slip into the listener role. Just this week, a friend asked me over lunch, "And when are we going to talk about you?" I laughed, because we probably aren't. I'd much rather hear about you.

Why do I love listening so much? People's stories are magic. Our stories are the tapestries that trail behind us like superhero cloaks. To listen is to examine the threads of those cloaks and find the nuance and sparkle in each one. To listen is to truly connect with someone. To feel heard is to feel valued. Listening is a gift to the listener and the storyteller.

Through listening, I've gotten to know some amazing people who otherwise would have been nameless and faceless strangers. I've met an Uber driver who was writing a pilot for Netflix, a security guard who marched with Dr. King, and an Irish missionary who'd spent a surprising amount of time exploring the Ozark mountains. In one particularly awe-inspiring encounter during a training at Kripalu's yoga retreat center, I stepped off an elevator and into the arms of a tiny, shuffling, 92-year old man with a thick European accent. "Will you walk with me?" he asked. Yes, of course. He unraveled for me the tapestry of his life, in which he survived the Holocaust in Estonia and came to America to study at the feet of a renowned guru for the next 40 years. He had dedicated his life to studying and teaching at Kripalu, then retired a few years before we met. "Now I spend my time walking the halls, talking to foxy women," he said. I laughed. What have you learned in all these years?, I asked, as we paced up and down the empty hallway. "Life is not so bad," he answered. "You just take things in stride and keep walking."

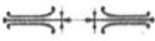

She thanks me again for letting her tell her sister's story.

"Now you know Hope," she says.

My breath catches. This always happens when I share a moment with strangers. There's always a tiny nugget of wisdom to tuck in a pocket in my heart and carry with me.

Now I know Hope. Both the person and the hope she had for her life. As well as her sister's hope that sharing her story might touch people in some way.

I hug her again. "Thank you for sharing your Hope with me."

We part ways, and I slip back into the festival crowd. I may never see her again, but I'm taking part of her with me. She has added another thread to my tapestry. A thread that glimmers with Hope.

CHAPTER 8

YES AND... NO

"It's aaallllllllll about acceptance, baby," she croons. Tears run from my eyes down my temples to my hair. I already know, but it feel good to hear her say it.

I'm lying on the floor of my yoga room. Beneath me is my great-grandmother's quilt and a beat-up old yoga mat. She's had her hands on me for over half an hour, giving me Reiki and guidance, calling on past-life memories and spirit guides. It's weird to some, but it works for me. It feels supportive and clarifying. I cry to release sadness. I tell her things I've only told a few close friends. Things I was ashamed to say out loud.

Acceptance is the mantra. She has me say over and over again, "I love and accept myself." Self-acceptance, acceptance of reality, accept, accept, accept. The word comes up over and over again.

"That's your theme," she says. "That's where your work is."

She has no idea how right she is.

⊰•⊱

The word "acceptance" gets thrown around a lot in spiritual and yogic communities. We are taught to accept our circumstances.

Our limitations. Our strengths. The people around us. That which we can control. That which we can't. And most importantly, ourselves, as the perfectly imperfect selves that we are.

I've always struggled with acceptance because I am, fundamentally, a fighter. I fight for what I believe in. I fight for those I love to be their best and most authentic selves. I fight to improve my circumstances and myself. On some level, I think I've rejected acceptance because it felt like giving into the status quo. I don't want to be okay with the now. I want to work for something bigger and better.

Acceptance has always been a troubling concept for me. So a couple of years ago, I sought an opportunity to confront my beliefs around acceptance.

I signed up for Improv classes.

Improv wasn't wildly out of my comfort zone. I've been an improv fan since I was a teenager and often go to shows. I did theater in high school and danced into my early twenties, so being on stage was nothing new. I was a little anxious about trying something different that I might not be "good" at right away, but I was mostly in it for the fun. I had no idea that it would challenge my some of my deepest-held beliefs.

The first two rules of improv are "Acceptance" and "Agreement." Basically, anything anyone says to you on stage, you accept as fact and build on. This drives the scene forward. So, if your scene partner says to you, "Doctor, the patient is here to see you," you would say, "Wonderful, he's here to have to new head sewn on," rather than, "I'm not a doctor; I'm a farmer!" Disagreement and rejection kill the momentum of the scene. Agreement and acceptance allow two or more people to tell a story together.

The application to life is obvious. In work settings, when a co-worker suggests an idea, rather than reject it right away, accept and add to it to foster feelings of support, teamwork, and brainstorming. In personal relationships, acceptance and agreement help your partner feel heard and create a sense of working together. In nearly every interaction you have with people, if you accept and agree, it will build the relationship and move things forward.

Great!

But wait, thought my poor, confused, therapy-filled brain. What about no? What about boundaries?

Sigh. And there I hit a wall.

So much of my personal work has been about learning to set boundaries. Having grown up in a household with few boundaries, I benefitted as an adult from 12 Step-inspired phrases like "'No' is a complete sentence" and "Appropriate boundaries create integrity." Boundaries help me feel empowered and in control. They give my life structure. They're hard sometimes, but they feel good.

And yet, I understand the principles of Acceptance and Agreement, too. Saying yes can lead to more excitement and adventure. Bigger and better projects. Deeper understanding and connection. And of course, saying yes to yourself--fully accepting and agreeing with the person that you are--is the essence of self-love.

So how does all this fit together? Can we agree and have boundaries at the same time? Can yes and no co-exist?

Carl Rogers said, "The curious paradox is that when I accept myself just as I am, then I can change." Bingo. Yes and no aren't opposites. Paradoxically, they work together. And when they do, profound change occurs.

No without yes is just rejection. It's often ego driven. It's saying, "I don't like this because I think it's wrong/it hurts me/I deserve better." It's reactive. It shuts down and creates more hurt.

But no can have a yes in front of it. "I see you for who you are, and I accept you for you and all that you are."

But here's the key… You can still say no after you accept.

"I accept you for who you are… and having you in my life isn't going to work for me right now."

"I accept that this job stressful and toxic… and I'm going to seek out something better for me."

"I accept that you need my help right now and value what I offer… and I'd love to help you some other time when it's a better fit for me."

Adding acceptance into boundaries, saying yes before saying no, makes communication more loving. It changes the dynamic on both sides. By accepting the situation and the person first, it also ensures that the boundary is well thought out, not reactive.

Yes and no can live together. And indeed, they must.

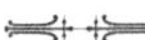

"You've done a lot of work," she says, almost in awe. "Like, really. Your spirit guides are telling me you've worked so hard. And it's okay now. You don't have to fight anymore. You can let your guard down." She keeps her hand on my back, so gentle and loving.

She can't know how deeply the words "fight" and "guard" resonate with me. I've been fighting my whole adult life, setting up walls to protect me, to claim the space that's mine. It's felt good. It's felt protective. It was the right thing at the time.

"You can be unguarded now," she says.

I'm protected enough. And even if I'm not, I'll be okay. Maybe it's finally time to give up the fight. To let the guards down. To trust.

Maybe it's time to just say yes.

CHAPTER 9

CALL IT A MIRACLE

"I don't really know how else to say it, but… They're telling me this is a miracle, what happened to you. It is a miracle."

I burst into tears. I know she's right. I've known in my gut all along. This thing I haven't been ready to fully process yet. It's a blessing. It's a gift. It was meant to be.

This is the truth I needed to hear. This is perspective I wanted permission to have on what was happening. I am so ready to finally embrace and celebrate it. I cry tears of joy.

The woman on the other end of the phone is Gabrielle Orr, a spiritual advisor to whom I've turned half a dozen times in recent years for guidance and comfort. She always reminds me of how loved I am. The "they" she refers to are the spirit guides who keep my Akashic records. They always tell me exactly what I need to hear. And this time, they're spot on.

The "miracle" I received is Herpes Simplex Virus 2, also known as genital herpes.

⬤

I knew what it was when I first saw the bump on my labia. It was a Tuesday morning in August, and I noticed it when I got up to use the bathroom. There it was, a small red spot on my right lip. I did what anyone in their right mind with an unknown spot on their genitals does: I panicked. I Googled. I convinced myself it was an ingrown hair or a reaction to my new body wash. But my gut knew what it was.

I was terrified.

Within two hours, thanks to an internet referral website, I had peed in a cup and given blood at a testing center. Two days later, the inconclusive results landed in my email inbox, with instructions to follow up with my gynecologist. More appointments, swabs, more waiting. The waiting was excruciating.

In the meantime, my body deteriorated. Most people know herpes by its skin symptoms, specifically bumps and lesions on the genitals and pelvis. Many don't realize that, for a small percentage of patients, a first herpes outbreak can cause debilitating, flu-like symptoms. I was in that unfortunate minority. My joints ached, especially below the waist. The lymph nodes on my bikini line swelled painfully to the point that walking became difficult. And the nausea. Oh my god, how my guts twisted, rejecting any thought of food. My pelvis burned like fire. I could barely get out of bed.

And finally, a diagnosis. After almost two full weeks of not knowing, my doctor finally called to let me know that I had tested positive for Herpes type 2, an incurable STD. I would have genital herpes for the rest of my life.

Unfortunately, the nightmare wasn't over. With all the pain in my pelvis in those two weeks, I had missed the symptoms of a urinary tract infection. By the time I made it to the emergency room, the infection had made its way to my kidneys, causing extreme pelvic and low back pain, and I could no longer walk unassisted. I had to be wheeled into the ER waiting room, where I proceeded to throw up before they could even ask my date of birth. I was given fluids and put on high dose antibiotics. I was told to be careful, to rest, to not work for a while. Between the herpes onset and the severe infection, my body had suffered a great shock.

The first round of antibiotics didn't work. So I was put on another. And another. I suffered persistent and debilitating UTIs for the better part of the next three months. In and out of doctor's offices: urgent care, gynecologist, urologist, back to urgent care. I spent most of my time in bed, unable to eat much more than toast. I nursed my pain and my nausea and prayed for relief.

Gradually, I began to feel a little better. Walking from the bedroom to the kitchen was no longer a slow, painful chore. I began teaching again, and by Halloween, I was able to go out with friends. My body slowly felt stronger, more normal.

As my body healed from the secondary infection and I felt a little more like myself, my mind and heart finally began to process the reality of my situation. I had herpes.

I had herpes.

One thing I knew for certain: I did not deserve this. I've always been incredibly careful around sex. I only have sex in the context of a monogamous, committed relationship, after "I love you"s have been exchanged. I pass no judgment on casual sex; it's just never been my thing. And even in my committed relationships, I always insisted on condoms. I did everything you're supposed to do.

And yet here I was, saddled with a stigmatizing diagnosis that would never, ever go away.

The emotional toll my herpes diagnosis took in those early months is hard to describe, and even worse than the physical toll the onset took on my body. As someone who had been hyper-responsible around sex, it pried at the very foundations about my beliefs about myself; I simply wasn't "the kind of person" who got herpes. I felt ashamed and dirty. Disgusting. I couldn't imagine telling anyone about my diagnosis. And the thought of being single and having to disclose my status to future potential partners made me physically ill. I felt like my life was over.

I cried so much. I mourned the loss of my "clean" status. I lamented about it in therapy, asking my therapists if anyone could ever love me.

Mostly, I hid.

I was so ashamed. When well-meaning friends and family asked me what was going on, why I had been sick for so long, I waved it off as "girl problems" and refused to answer their questions. The stigma felt so heavy. In doing internet research on my new status, I found out that herpes is considered the most highly stigmatized STD in the world, even more so than HIV, as patients with HIV and AIDS are labeled "survivors" and considered "brave" for disclosing their status. Patients with herpes, on the other hand, are almost universally thought of dirty, slutty, and unclean. And dating with herpes presents a world of complications. On some surveys, single people say they're more likely to reject a potential partner for having herpes than they are for having a felony criminal record. Herpes is largely feared and reviled in our collective consciousness.

But this universal stigma ignores how incredibly common and relatively benign herpes actually is. The CDC estimates that 1 in 5 sexually active adults has herpes simplex virus, with many unaware that they have it, as it can be asymptomatic--but still contagious--especially in men. And while the first outbreak can be painful and complicated for some, as it was for me, the virus itself causes little more than a chronic skin condition, which can be easily and effectively managed with daily medication. Safe sex practices greatly reduce the risk of transmission from one partner to another, and many people with herpes report that--once they worked through the shame and stigma--their status has caused them to communicate more openly and honestly with their partners, which can ultimately lead to greater intimacy and sexual satisfaction.

And yet, the stigma persists. Many people report feeling un-loveable and tainted after their diagnosis, as I did, and some even consider suicide. Resources for patients with herpes outside of a doctor's office are slim, and herpes support groups are all but non-existent due in no small part to those persistent feelings of shame. (Who wants to be seen walking into a herpes support group?) In recent years, a handful of activists have called for "shout your status" campaigns on social media, but they've yet to take off in a major way, as people fear bullying or rejection after disclosure.

It's easy to feel helpless and hopeless after a herpes diagnosis. I did for many, many months after mine. But ultimately, I was ready to let go of the shame. I called Gabrielle, hoping for permission to take a different perspective on what life with herpes would look like.

And she delivered. As soon as she said the word "miracle," I knew. I knew exactly what life with herpes would look like for me and, more importantly, how I could free myself of the shame.

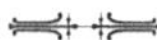

I went on medication right away after my diagnosis and have been on it ever since. I take the highest daily dose of viral suppressant, and fortunately, I've been outbreak-free since those initial terrifying months. As long as I stay on suppressant medication and use condoms every time I have sex, my chance of passing on the virus to my partners is close to zero.

There are days I'm still angry at the man who gave me herpes. He had it for years without knowing. He neglected to get tested and unknowingly spread the virus to me. In my darkest moments, I blame him. But in my lighter, more conscious moments, I see things very differently.

For some reason, this virus showed up in my body. It chose me. I will never be free of it. We will live together in the same space until the day I die. And so, my only choice is to be a good host. Rejecting it and hiding it serves neither of us and does nothing to relieve my shame. And so, I will make the more loving choice with this viral guest. I will care for myself and the body that is now its home. I will get enough sleep and eat well and do yoga every day. I will take care of both of us.

And rather than live in shame, I will use acceptance of us both--me and the virus--as the metric against which I measure all love in the future. Whoever loves me will have to love us both, will have to welcome both of us into their life. This virus and me, we are a package deal now; there is no changing that. And the man who gets to love me for life will have a heart big enough for both of us.

On the phone that day, over a year after my initial diagnosis, Gabrielle assured me that this virus will ensure that only people of the highest vibration with the purest hearts will enter my life from now on. Only people who will see me for me and have my best interest at heart. She told me over and over that I have no reason to be ashamed. "This is not something to hide," she said. "This is sacred information you will share with people. It's not a secret. It's sacred."

And so that is how I choose to see this virus that chose me: It is sacred. I am in holy communion with a microscopic organism that lives on the nerve endings in my pelvis. Sometimes I rest my hands on my lower belly and wish it well. I hope you are happy here, I say. I hope my body is a good home for you. Lovingkindness erases the anger, fear, and pain.

One thing I have come to know for certain: This diagnosis does not define me. It doesn't make me any less loveable or worthy. I am not perfect in this acceptance. Even as I write this, my hands are shaking at the thought of disclosing my status in writing. But I can't let that fear dictate my actions. Shame thrives in silence, and I'm done with shame. I am prepared for any judgment that might be directed my way due to people knowing I have herpes. And I am prepared to release it and love myself all the more.

Prior to contracting herpes, I was terrified of getting an STD. I wasn't sure how I would cope if I did. That morning in August when I woke up with a bump on my labia forced me to face that fear. The Universe asked me that day, "Can you love and accept yourself even now?" And I have learned that the answer is yes. I can love myself, and I can love this passenger who will ride around with me for the rest of my days. My love and acceptance only grows in its presence.

And so, for this miracle, I give thanks. And for all the miracles that showed up in the guise of tragedies, I give thanks. And for all the future miracles that will show up shrouded in fear and pain, I pray only for the discernment and wisdom to be able to lift the veil and see the lessons of love there, just beneath, ready to show us how truly infinite our hearts can be.

CHAPTER 10

BORN TO DO THIS

"I am not afraid. I was born to do this."

- Joan of Arc

I take my shoes off and run toward the water, clutching my long skirt in one hand, still giddy and laughing from the golf cart ride that got me here. My hair is tangled from whipping around my face as a flew down the highway, cars honking at me as I took the sharp turn up the gravel path that led me to the beach. My glee is childlike.

I'm in Colonia del Sacramento, Uruguay, plunging my bare feet into the waters of the Rio de la Plata. Across the river is Buenos Aires, where I have been for the last week. I feel very far from home, and the distance is exhilarating.

I came here alone. I bought the ticket with money I made doing the thing I love most in the world. I've chased this solo adventure, navigated travel and sightseeing in a country where I don't speak the language, mostly just to prove to myself that I can. I wasn't sure exactly why I needed this trip so badly, only that I did, that it was necessary, and that I would know the reason once I got there.

Here on a beach in a tiny, sleepy town in Uruguay, I find the answer.

I've come a long way to get here, literally and figuratively. I'm 34, in the middle of decade of life that I'm hell-bent on defining for myself, free from the judgments and expectations others might place on me. I'm chasing a dream of travel and teaching that continues to evolve, and becomes more beautiful and fulfilling the more I open my heart to it. I've survived trauma and betrayal and lived to tell the tales and, on my good days, been able to help others struggling with the same issues. I've accepted that I'm a woman living with herpes, and I love myself and the viral passenger that's joined me on the ride of my life. And I've learned with great certainty that I don't need a man in my life to complete me, that I'm thoroughly complete and worthy all on my own.

Much like my early days, life in recent years has been defined by movement: leapfrogging from one crisis to another, flying through the air on nothing but faith, and chasing a life of travel. There are times when I feel like I never stopping moving, never stop running, never stop putting one foot in front of the other.

It's taken a lot to get me here--hours of therapy, buckets of tears, a million yoga poses, a lot of prayer and meditation, two plane rides, one Uber, a ferry, and a rickety gas-powered golf cart--but here on a deserted beach in Uruguay, it all comes together. In this moment, in spite of and because of all of it, I am simply happy.

The wind whips my skirt around my bare legs. Waves lap at my ankles. For a few glorious moments, I have the beach all to myself. The solitude is breathtaking. I turn my face toward the sun, smile, and offer up a simple prayer of gratitude.

I feel the weight of all it took to get me here fall away. I remember the lesson I learned so long ago when I laid down on my first yoga mat in that tiny studio in Tuscaloosa:

Sometimes, all you really need is to just be still.

CHAPTER 11

STILL WRITING

This is not the end of my story.

It is the middle.

My story didn't end when I was raped at 19. It didn't end when I finally beat my eating disorder at 24. It didn't end when I got divorced at 30. It didn't end when I was diagnosed with a disease I didn't ask for at 32. And it didn't end in that exquisitely joyful moment on a beach in Uruguay at 34.

It's not even close to over.

The women in my recovery community say often, "My story is still being written." I tell my teacher trainees, "Assume you're in the middle." One of my counseling mentors says, "More will be revealed." However you say it, the story isn't finite; it continues.

This is simply a pause. A breath. A moment between, before the next pose, the next transition, the next big thing.

I finally wrote that book I always dreamed of. But this is only the first part of my story. I have a lot more to say. I'll keep writing. I'll keep telling stories. I'll keep living out loud--seeking travel and yoga and the holy assignments of blessedly human relationships--so I have more stories to tell.

My story is still being written.

And I can't wait to see what happens next.

CONCLUSION: YOU'RE STRONGER THAN YOU THINK YOU ARE

I don't remember where I was when I first said the words, "You're stronger than you think you are," but I remember the thunder in my belly as the words left my mouth. I knew that I had found a Truth, far bigger than just me. I knew I had to say it, and keep saying it.

As I started sharing it in my classes--dropping it at just the right moment during a long-held, challenging pose--the statement seemed to resonate with my students, as well. Its echo returned to me, showing me the ripples this deep Truth made. Students began to say it back to me with a smile. They told me they said it to themselves during hard times. One student even told me that her children started saying it to themselves when they were struggling to complete a task. I realized I was on to something.

When I connected with my teacher, Sadie Nardini, she encouraged us to find our Core Message, which she defined as that one sentence that's central to your yoga teaching. As soon as she explained the idea, I knew that I already had my Core Message. I'd been saying it for years, both to myself and my students. It was and is a hard-won belief from years of fighting my own demons and coming out the other side in a place of hope and healing. It's the lesson the Universe has been trying to teach me all along.

You're stronger than you think you are.

This is the wisdom I was given to share. It is the sound of my heartbeat, the rhythm of my breath, and the pulse in my veins. It is the thing I can say when no other words come. I will whisper it, say it, shout it every day, because I must. It is the one thing that radiates out of me. There is no other Truth for me but this Truth.

And because it was given to me, I have an obligation to share it. In every interaction I have, it is the undercurrent. When I celebrate my friends' successes, you're stronger than you think you are. When my yoga students look at me like I'm crazy for suggesting a challenging yoga pose, you're stronger than you think you are. When my trainees doubt their ability to stand up and use their voices to teach, you're stronger than you think you are.

There are times I want to run up to strangers in the street, grab them by the shoulders, and say, "Don't you see? This is your truth. You are Divine and powerful. You are so much more than your give yourself credit for. Please recognize your strength as I do and join me in celebrating it!"

What I love most about this message is its recursive infiniteness. It is a statement without end. You know how strong you think you are now? You're stronger than that. And when you internalize that next level of strength, you must pause to recognize that you are stronger still. And stronger beyond that, and beyond that. And on and on and on. It is the lesson we never stop learning.

And so I'll keep saying it, because I keep hearing it in my own life, over and over, after every new challenge I face. My rape taught me that I'm stronger than I think I am in using my own voice, setting boundaries, and healing from trauma. Every break-up I've been through has taught me that I'm stronger than I think I am in standing on my own, taking care of myself, and moving through grief. And my most recent health crisis has taught me that I'm stronger than I think I am in facing a stigmatized diagnosis, not buying into self-esteem-destroying myths, and honoring my true worth as a loved and lovable person.

I must have learned these lessons for a reason. They cannot exist solely for my benefit. These must be stories I'm meant to tell. These must be teachings I'm meant to share. I have to send these lessons out into the world in hopes that they will benefit someone else.

And so I tell you--yes, You, holding this book, my sweet friend--you must know this one thing to be true: You're stronger than you think you are. Your history proves this; you've come through so much to get to this point and survived every bit of it. Your story is inspiring. And whatever is coming at you now or will come at you in the future, you will survive that and inspire even more. And you are never alone. Even when it seems like there's no one there, you are in the company of the immense, abiding strength inside you. You have you, and you need no one else.

There is freedom in this truth. If you can learn to trust it, then you know that there's nothing you can't handle and no dream you can't chase. Your life can be as big and bold as you wish for it to be, and then you can wish on even more.

I hope you already believe this about yourself. But in case you don't, I'm going to keep saying it. I will send this vibration out into the Universe, in hopes that it makes contact with the hearts of those who need it. No matter where I go, what I do, or what challenges I overcome, these will be the words on my lips.

It is my belief, my mantra, and my offering to you.

You're so much stronger than you think you are.

ACKNOWLEDGMENTS

First, foremost, and always, I have to send immense gratitude my teachers--Dolly Stavros and Sadie Nardini--who lit the way forward. I wouldn't be the person or teacher I am today without you. My gratitude for you is never-ending.

Second, to my family. My brother Ben for being my favorite person and indulging my wacky Christmas picture ideas. My Dad for the love of a good story. And my Mom for the gift of writing.

To my beloved Connie. The Frack to my Frick, my sister-from-another-mister, my daily reminder that I am loved and needed. I don't know what I'd do without you.

To Kim, my wise yoga mama, who calms me and reminds me just how hard I kick ass.

To Jacob, the Libertine to my Bon Vivant. I can't wait to get kicked out of the nursing home together when we're old.

To Carla Jean Whitley for her friendship, guidance, wisdom, inspiration, and editing genius. She's thanked me by name in two books so far, so I owe her at least one more. Although probably a lot more than that.

To Javacia Harris Bowser who shepherded this book to fruition. Your talent, dedication, and drive are rivaled only by Beyonce. This book truly is yours, too.

To Josh Parker for the beautiful cover image for this book and the many years of laughter and friendship.

To all the members of my yoga community in Birmingham who have inspired and supported me along the way: Nancy Rhodes, Jasper Elliott Wolfe, Shannon Andrews Skipper, Annie Damsky, Stephen Fletcher, Emilie Maynor, Kim Drye, Pilar Taylor, and many others.

To the women in my recovery community. Oh my God, what would I do without you? Thank you for the daily reminders that I'm sane, whole, loveable, and loved.

To the women who shared their wisdom about writing, publishing, and body positivity, all of which made me a much better writer: Amy Bickers, Stephanie Naman, Jennifer King, and Mary-Berkeley Gaines.

To Mollie Erickson and Kara Dye for invaluable feedback and encouragement.

To the women in my writing communities, especially all the members of See Jane Write who inspired and supported me during the writing of this book.

To the women who gave me the gift of mental health, so that I can in turn help others: Dr. Barbara Johnson, Susan Hart, Diane Reid, Beebe Roberts, and Dr. Misty Smith.

To my many, many friends who always make me laugh and pick me up when I'm down. There are too many to list here by name, but please know that if you're reading this and wondering, "Does she means me?"... Yeah, I absolutely do. I'm forever grateful for my Tribe.

To my wonderful cats. Murray--whose time on earth came to an end during the writing of this book--for his great, big heart. And Montana for being love incarnate, my little furry soul mate.

To my person, for walking this long and difficult road with me.

To my yoga students, for giving me a reason to be.

And finally, to the extraordinary human beings who have chosen me to lead them through teacher training. I can't even start to write about you without getting teary-eyed. You are, without a doubt, the single greatest blessing in my entire life. You have taught me more than I could ever possibly teach you, and you remind me every day of the extraordinary power of the human spirit. I love you, I love you, I love you.

ABOUT THE AUTHOR

Melissa Scott is a yoga teacher, therapist, and writer based in Birmingham, Alabama. She writes and presents regularly on yoga, feminism, and body-positivity. She leads yoga teacher trainings and workshops both at home and around the country. She enjoys spending time with her two cats and drinking lots of kombucha. This is her first book.

www.MelissaScottYoga.com

www.ingramcontent.com/pod-product-compliance
Lightning Source LLC
Chambersburg PA
CBHW070830260726
48654CB00025B/793